Regulating Reproduction

ROBERT H. BLANK

REGULATING
REPRODUCTION

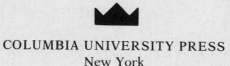

COLUMBIA UNIVERSITY PRESS
New York

COLUMBIA UNIVERSITY PRESS
New York

Columbia University Press
New York   Oxford
Copyright © 1990 Columbia University Press
All rights reserved

Library of Congress Cataloging-in-Publication Data
Blank, Robert H.
Regulating reproduction / Robert H. Blank.
p. cm.
Includes bibliographical references.
ISBN 0-231-07016-0
1. Human reproductive technology—Social aspects.
I. Title.
RG133.5.B58 1990 176—dc20 89-77670
CIP

Casebound editions of Columbia University Press books are Smyth-sewn
and printed on permanent and durable acid-free paper

Printed in the United States of America
c 10 9 8 7 6 5 4 3 2 1

To
Margaret Bremner Scott
and the memory of
James Donald Scott

CONTENTS

PREFACE

W E CURRENTLY are in the midst of a revolution in human reproduction. The rapid proliferation of an array of human genetic and reproductive technologies over the last decade deeply challenges traditional values regarding procreation and threatens to undermine fundamental social structures. These new capabilities intervene at the most basic levels of human existence and create increasingly difficult dilemmas regarding if and when to exercise these new-found powers.

This book focuses attention on the political context of human reproduction and on the excruciating public policy issues accompanying these remarkable reproductive innovations. Although a considerable literature exists on the ethical issues surrounding reproductive technologies, to date the policy dimensions have been obscured. Also, many books on this subject are primarily technical in nature or center on a specific application. In contrast, this book provides an overview of the cumulative impact on society of a wide array of new intervention techniques and of the social patterns that accompany or precede their use. It also provides a critical analysis of political activity both in the United States and other countries.

As the title indicates, this book places emphasis on the need to regulate these emerging capabilities in order to maximize the benefits they promise but minimize the problems they create. I argue for the urgent necessity of a rigorous national dialogue on social priorities regarding human procreation. Collectively, we must decide how we desire to handle the reproductive revolution and deal with the volatile and divisive policy issues that accompany it. To do so, we must place considerably more emphasis on our responsibility to future generations and make a renewed effort to reach a consensus, wherever possible, on how best to resolve the challenges we increasingly face.

Although our options at present are virtually unbounded, the rapid expansion of our ability to intervene in human procreation is closing those very alternatives which traditionally we have embraced. No longer is human life the product solely of natural happenings, fate, or even manipulation of the environment. We now hold the keys to direct intervention in the most fundamental aspects of human life. However, as we acquire the capacity to control and direct the human condition we also assume an awesome responsibility, whether willingly or not, for the choices we make.

ACKNOWLEDGMENTS

ALTHOUGH MANY individuals have had an impact on this book, the contributions of a few warrant special acknowledgment. The book was strengthened considerably by the valuable suggestions of Lori Andrews and Andrea Bonnicksen. Their thoughtful, critical reviews of earlier drafts of the manuscript forced me to address with more clarity some of the more difficult conceptual problems surrounding human reproduction. Kate Wittenberg's editorial encouragement and Leslie Bialler's expert computer production skills were crucial to completion of the book. I also thank Carolyn Cradduck and other staff members of the Program for Biosocial Research at Northern Illinois University for their work on the manuscript and Mike Adams, who as my graduate assistant, spent innumerable hours in the library tracking down sources. Although the book is substantially stronger because of their contributions, any remaining shortcomings are my responsibility and should not reflect on any of these persons.

Finally, I want to thank my wife, Mallory, and my children, Jeremy, Mai-Ling, and Maigin for their cooperation and patience. They have apparently survived yet another book project.

Regulating Reproduction

CHAPTER ONE

The Changing Context of Human Reproduction

*I*N AUSTRALIA, a sixteen-month-old girl greets her recently newborn twin, the product of in vitro fertilization using an embryo frozen for two years. In Tennessee a divorced couple go to
court over custody of seven frozen embryos—she calls the embryos
the "beginning of life" and her only chance at bearing a child,
while he fights to keep the embryos frozen, at least for the present.
In South Africa, a grandmother gives birth to her grandchildren
that she carried as a surrogate mother for her daughter. In a highly
publicized case, the New Jersey Supreme Court reverses a trial
court's ruling that surrogate mother contracts are enforceable. In
California, a lesbian who had physically inseminated her lover
with donor sperm sues for "paternity" rights (and loses) when the
couple splits up. In Massachusetts, a law is passed requiring insurance carriers to pay for in vitro fertilization and other reproductive

1

technologies for infertile couples. In San Diego, a woman is charged with child abuse for harming, by drug abuse, the fetus she is carrying. Meanwhile, in Washington, D.C., a caesarean section is performed on a dying, 26 weeks pregnant, cancer patient against her expressed wishes. This is done supposedly for the benefit of the child, who dies upon delivery.

Hardly a day passes without reports of similar instances in which common assumptions concerning human reproduction are challenged. There is no doubt that one of the most dramatic and poignant areas of change in the last decades of the twentieth century centers on this most fundamental level of human life—procreation of our future. The way we approach this future will very much depend on how we deal with the rapidly expanding array of reproductive technologies and services that are now emerging. The policy issues that follow these technical changes are bound to be among the most problematic we have ever faced. Their resolution is bound to require considerably more commitment and effort than has been forthcoming. The failure now to address these issues head on, however, will require even more difficult policy decisions in the near future.

REPRODUCTIVE CHOICE IN THE UNITED STATES

In every society, few areas of human intervention are as sensitive or engender as much intense debate as those relating to human reproduction. According to Ribes (1978:114), this is not surprising since the whole existence of the living is organized for reproduction. Although some limits are placed on procreative choice in almost every society, in most western societies procreation is viewed as a fundamental right inherent in the very survival of the individual. The United Nations Universal Declaration of Human Rights (1948), for instance, emphasizes the right to marry and found a family, free from constraint, and affords special care and assistance to motherhood. According to Article 16, the family is the natural and fundamental unit of society and entitled to protection by the state. Reproductive choice, in an absolute sense, is seen as an essential human right.

In the United States, procreative rights are viewed as fundamental human rights. For instance, Justice William O. Douglas in *Skinner v. Oklahoma* (1942) applied the concept of "fundamental interests" to procreation when he placed compulsory sterilization within the confines of the equal protection clause of the Fourteenth Amendment: "We are dealing here with legislation which involves one of the basic civil rights of man. Marriage and procreation are fundamental to the very existence and survival of the race. The power to sterilize, if exercised, may have subtle, far reaching and devastating effects. . .there is no redemption for the individual whom the law touches. . . . He is forever deprived of a basic liberty."

Since *Skinner*, the constitutional status of reproductive choice has been expanded. Justice Goldberg in a concurring opinion in *Griswold v. Connecticut* (1965) sees the marital relationship as a fundamental area of privacy protected by the Ninth Amendment. The state can interfere with marriage and procreation only upon proof of a "compelling state interest." This philosophy was reiterated in *Roe v. Wade* (1973) where the Court ruled that a state cannot dictate to a pregnant woman whether or not she may have an abortion during the first trimester of pregnancy and in *Eisenstadt v. Baird* (1972) where the Court recognized "the right of the individual, married or single, to be free of unwarranted government intrusion into matters so fundamentally affecting a person as the decision whether to bear or beget a child."

Wald (1975:4) argues that rights as important to human existence as the right to bear and raise children and to sexual freedom, in or outside of marriage, should not be denied to any human except under extraordinary circumstances. She asserts that "every human being should be presumed to have these rights unless someone can show an almost certain probability of disastrous consequences" if they are exercised. Ramsey (1975:238) contends that "parenthood is certainly one of those courses of action natural to man, which cannot without violation be disassembled and put together again. . ." Similarly, Murphy and associates (1978:367) conclude that there must be a "presumption in favor of the parents to reproduce" as they desire. The state may interfere only if parents abuse their privileges, but at present there is no "justification for restricting this right by law or even social pressure."

Lappé (1972:420) is disturbed by the current advocacy of societal intervention in childbearing decisions, the denial of medical care to the congenitally damaged, and the sterilization of carriers. He contends that society has no right to intervene in childbearing decisions except in very rare circumstances. Despite acknowledgement of statistics on social costs, Lappé (1972:425) states: "I know of no such decision. . .where the decision to procreate or bear children should be the choice of other than the parents." Although Milunsky (1977:185) reiterates that a child has a right to begin life with a sound mind and body, still he contends that, ultimately, the parents should have the right to make the final decision.

In contrast, other observers argue that even if procreation is an inalienable right, it can be regulated by a society which is concerned with the existence of the child to be born and its own survival as a society. Reproduction in these terms is a right shared with society as a whole and is but part of a larger complex of rights, responsibilities, and obligations. For instance, while Ribes (1978:118) admits procreation is a fundamental human right, he concludes that this right cannot be exercised without "due respect for the vital requirements of the child to be born and those of society." Although most persons with this perspective agree that procreation is a fundamental human right, they contend that it must be weighed against broader social concerns. Etzioni (1974:51) expresses concern for individual rights, but he sees the tendency to give the individual "unlimited priority" over society to be counterproductive, because "the individual is part of society and needs it for his or her survival and well-being."

Likewise, Reilly (1977:132) asserts that no rights are absolute and that it is erroneous to conclude that state action to control reproduction on genetic grounds could never survive a constitutional challenge. He concludes (148) on a cautious note, however: "The right to marry and the right to bear children are so fundamental that a heavy burden of proof should be placed on those who claim that society should give special priority to the reduction of genetic disease. . . . I would demand a convincing demonstration that a really impressive societal benefit could be derived from more intrusive programs." Although many individuals would impose some restraints on procreative rights in order to protect affected children, others take an even stronger stand for societal intervention in reproductive choice. For instance, a strict utilitarian approach such as Fletcher's (1974) "situational ethics" gives society wide discretion in reproductive matters if circumstances warrant intrusion in order to achieve the greatest good. Fletcher contends that one must compute gains and losses following several courses of action or nonaction and then select that alternative which offers the most good despite its implication for individual rights. The common welfare must be safeguarded, by compulsory state control if necessary. Bentley Glass (1975:56–57) agrees that advances in human genetics result in a reordered priority of rights. Changes in technology demand that the right of individuals to procreate must give way to a more "paramount" right—"the right of every child to enter life with an adequate physical and mental endowment."

THE PROCESS OF REPRODUCTION

Reproduction is more than simply a biological event. Instead, it is a complex activity that develops over time and involves a series of disparate though interrelated behaviors. It is a process of major social significance for the family and, in the aggregate, for society. Its importance emanates from the genetic, biological, and social experiences that comprise it. Until very recently, these aspects were intractably joined. Although questions of paternity often were raised, maternity was certain. Only when the "mother" (genetic and gestation) "gave up" her baby for adoption was ambiguity introduced, and here the law stepped in to clarify "legal parent-hood." Still, difficult legal dilemmas arose when a "natural mother" changed her mind and demanded custody of her child from the adoptive parents.

For Robertson (1983:408), claims of procreative freedom logi-cally extend to three components of reproduction: conception, ges-tation and labor, and childrearing. Although these aspects "com-bine to create a powerful experience," each of them has independent personal value and meaning. Attention has focused only recently on the biological experience of bearing and giving birth as aspects of procreative freedom. Childrearing is a fulfilling experience de-serving respect, whether or not the person who raises also provided genes or bore the child. There is a tendency today to deal almost exclusively on reproductive choices about who may conceive, bear, and rear a child, with a clear emphasis on the woman's rights to avoid pregnancy. These choices, however, are distinct from choices about the conduct that occurs in the process of conceiving, bearing, and rearing.

Considerable effort is needed to clarify this critical expansion of the notion of procreative rights, especially in light of recent ad-vances in genetics and medicine. No longer is the genetic linkage unambiguous. Virtually any kind of combination of germ material is now possible. Artificial insemination, in vitro fertilization, and various embryo transfer techniques are displacing the traditional premise that the woman who conceives the child, bears it and raises it. In other words, the process of procreation itself is undergoing continuous change. Therefore, it is dangerous to focus too closely on one predominant procreative right at the exclusion of others. For instance, by stressing the right of one woman to terminate pregnancy through abortion, we may be voiding the right of another woman to adopt that potential child and fulfill her freedom to rear a child she biologically cannot conceive or bear.

THE FIRST REVOLUTION: REMOVING REPRODUCTION FROM SEX

The first revolution in reproduction was the separation of procreation from sexual intercourse made possible by the availability of safe and effective contraceptive techniques. Sexual intercourse no longer led to reproduction; it could now be undertaken as an independent activity without the actuality or fear of pregnancy. The development of the birth control pill and intrauterine devices, and their widespread use since the 1960s, undisputedly have had a revolutionary impact on our society. According to Snowden and associates (1983:5), the distinction of sex from reproduction has "inexorably altered the relationship between men and women, and husbands and wives, in ways that are only now becoming apparent."

In the past, most attempts by societies to control reproduction were based on the assumption that sexual intercourse led to procreation. By controlling who was permitted to have sexual intercourse, reproduction could be channeled into societally approved modes. Thus, incest laws were designed less to protect young girls from violation of a sexual nature than to prevent the reproduction of children with genetic anomalies. Consanguineous marriages, likewise, were legislated against on the premise that the offspring produced would be a burden to society. The current availability of effective sterilization techniques undercuts the genetic dimension of laws against consanguineous marriages. Also, by separating sex from reproduction, legal constraints on the age of consent and social pressures to limit the number of progeny take on a new significance. Without the risk of pregnancy and the birth of a child, sexual intercourse has become a private and personal activity between the participants. Consequently, justification for government involvement is more difficult to achieve.

The diffusion of contraception technologies across western societies also altered the concept of reproductive responsibility and was accompanied by an explicit emphasis on population control. Although the fear of overpopulation has moderated since the 1960s, the premise that we must keep population growth within manageable bounds is widely accepted. This, in turn, has contributed to a concern for quality of life of those children brought into the world. Among many elements in society, people with large families are viewed as socially irresponsible, and prolific parents are criticized. Moreover, "many concerned parents are carefully planning for children, and because of perceived social expectation and pressure to produce a limited number of children, there is an increasing parental concern for the genetic health of each child." (Twiss 1974:235)

As the family size decreases, it is natural that parents will be more willing to utilize available technologies so that they might have the healthiest and "best" one or two children possible. This attitude pattern will likely increase demand for an even broader array of reproductive innovations.

Social forces reflect the general economic context as well. As the United States faces a probable drop in standard of living and resources become even more exiguous, reproductive intervention programs will receive considerably more attention and public support. In the past, even in times of abundant resources, those affected by genetic disorders and other unfortunate persons have received minimal support. In times of scarce resources, it is likely that those at the bottom will be the targets of cost saving efforts and increasingly will be seen as burdens to society. Greater pressures to reduce this burden are readily translated into support for programs aimed at eliminating the problem and reducing the number of those persons affected and for technologies that help assure propagation of healthy children.

A reinforcing trend, which Charles Frankel (1976:24) sees as contributing toward a growing tolerance of reproductive intervention, is the decline of the family and of the "marital idea." Kass (1971:784) argues that the breakdown of the family threatens to destroy our sense of continuity with the past and the future, since it is the family through which we acquire links with the past, as well as a sense of commitment to the future. He sees this trend as

contributing to the depersonalization of society. Parenthood now
has much less meaning than in past generations. The acceptance of
new lifestyles has provided alternatives to the traditional family,
while the high divorce rates complicate the notion of family. Overall, changing values regarding the centrality of the family to human existence have contributed to an atmosphere where conventional parent-child relationships are defined largely from an
individualistic perspective.

Although these contextual factors together appear to provide a
favorable social framework for the development of reproductive
intervention programs, their presence does not ensure implementation. Countering these trends are values relating to the dignity of
the person and to self-determination which are central to American
culture. Despite the social trends summarized above and the wide
discrepancies in distribution of goods and services, the liberal value
system still reflects a concern for the human as something special.
The extent to which these current social patterns accelerate the
"erosion of the idea of man as something splendid or divine" (Kass
1971), and replace it with the view that human beings are not
unique but something to be manipulated genetically, will depend
in large part on how the issues are presented to the public and
what technological possibilities become reality.

THE SECOND REVOLUTION: REMOVING SEX
FROM REPRODUCTION

We are now quickly entering the second revolution in reproduction,
which promises to be accompanied by severe alterations in social
attitudes and behavior that exceed those changes, still reverberat-
ing, caused by the first revolution. Precipitating this revolution is
the aggregation of reproduction technologies that effectively removes the need for sexual intercourse from reproduction. Artificial
insemination, in vitro fertilization, embryo transfer, cryopreservation techniques, and a host of imminent innovations allow for
many combinations of human germ material without sexual intercourse. The impact of these technologies on a variety of social
structures, both values and institutions, is considerable. Most
prominent are their ramifications on conventional notions of the
family, parenthood, and procreative autonomy. Inherent in these
alterations are essential reevaluations of relationships among men

and women in society. Although the specific techniques vary substantially, the one feature they have in common is that they effectively segregate reproduction from sexual intercourse.

Each of these technologies raises serious challenges to conventional family structuring and other social institutions we have long taken as given. Critical to the concept of family has been parenthood. Although recent trends have increased the number of purposively childless couples, facilitated by effective fertility control technologies, parenthood remains a central aspect of family life. Until recently, parenthood was largely an uncomplicated term referring to the couple that conceived and raised the child. Legal procedures were established for those instances where the parents of conception surrendered custody of the baby to the adoptive parents. Other exceptions were limited by biological constraints which linked conception, childbearing, and childrearing.

The rapid diffusion of the array of reproductive-aiding technologies dramatically eliminates the biological restraints on human procreation, and thus threatens the traditional assumptions of parenthood. They compel redefinition of the terms "mother" and "father" and complicate the roles played by various actors in the procreative process. Unfortunately, terms traditionally used to describe participants in the entire procreative process are no longer relevant in light of the technological advances in human reproduction that allow us to subdivide what was once assumed to be a single process.

Motherhood

Generally, motherhood has included the production of the ovum, childbearing, and childrearing. The "mother" of a child produced the egg containing her genetic material, carried to term the product of fertilization through sexual intercourse, and raised the child to adulthood. With the introduction of human reproduction intervention technologies, it is possible that each of these three processes be performed by a different woman. The *genetic mother* is the woman who supplies the egg to be fertilized by in vitro fertilization or the embryo for transfer. She might or might not be the *carrying mother* in whose womb the embryo implants and develops to term. Finally, the *nurturing mother* is the woman who cares for the baby once it is born. Snowden and associates (1983:32) call the woman who fulfills all three roles the *complete mother*. In addition to these singular or total roles, reproductive technologies permit three combinations: genetic-carrying mother, genetic-nurturing mother, and carrying-nurturing mother. Potential egg fusion and gene splicing technologies in the future might require more precise distinctions within genetic motherhood and the fetal transfer possibilities within carrying motherhood.

Fatherhood

Likewise, the definition of fatherhood must be clarified within the context of this reproductive revolution. The male is involved in two processes: production and delivery of the sperm and nurturing the child after birth. Artificial insemination, in combination with cryopreservation, separates these two processes and forces us to distinguish between the *genetic father* who provides the sperm for either internal or external fertilization, and the *nurturing father* who cares for the child after birth, but who has not supplied the genetic material during fertilization. The nurturing father takes on responsibility for raising the child and often is the husband of the complete mother, who has undergone artificial insemination. The *complete father*, according to Snowden et al. (1983:35), is the man who performs both singular roles. In many cases, the genetic father is an anonymous sperm donor or one of several men whose semen have been mixed prior to insemination.

Implications for Defining Parenthood

The changing definitions of motherhood and fatherhood have introduced many legal and moral dilemmas and complicated the once explicit notion of parenthood. Potentially, a child could have five or more parents, not counting stepparents. This raises important questions concerning the rights and responsibilities inherent in each parental role and over which role takes precedence. For instance, does the genetic mother retain any control over her germ material once it is implanted in a carrying mother? In most societies, all three roles of motherhood have long been interrelated components. By separating them, these technologies necessitate clarification of the relative importance of each component. This ambiguity in parenthood also raises problems for the children produced through these methods, because most cultures have assumed that each person has a past in terms of family history as well as a present in terms of a current family relationship.

The special relationship that constitutes a family is important both for the individual and as a basic unit of social organization. Through the family, individuals acquire basic values, roles, and trust. Although recent socialization research indicates that families share with other agents the shaping of children's views of the world, they remain critical to the maintenance of society. The most important function of the family is its role as the primary reproductive unit. Therefore, it is crucial that ambiguities in parenthood introduced by reproductive technologies be diminished through efforts to specify what roles take precedence.

TECHNOLOGY-MEDIATED REPRODUCTION

It has become commonplace in the literature to use the term "artificial reproduction" to describe procreation which is achieved through the use of these new technologies. This term is a loaded one, in that it creates a false dichotomy by labeling reproduction via sexual intercourse as natural and everything else as artificial. Traditional assumptions of what is normal are constantly being challenged in all areas of human endeavor. For instance, the definition of death is consistently undergoing transformation as we move to more and more precise concepts of brain death. Although nontraditional approaches circumvent what conventionally is the normal reproduction process and often separate it from sexual intercourse, it is likely that in time they very well might be the normal means of procreation.

The term "technology-mediated" reproduction is a more accurate representation of these new methods of reproduction. Other appropriate terms are technology-aided or technology-assisted procreation. Although these terms are more unwieldly than is artificial reproduction, they are more nearly neutral and more accurate. For consistency, technology-mediated reproduction (TMR) will be used here to refer to the aggregation of techniques that together constitute human reproduction technologies.

The availability of technology-mediated methods of conception complicates what it means to have a personal identity. Just as the

children of a *Brave New World* (Huxley 1946) have no identifiable
parents, a notion Plato embraced for the Guardians, so there continues to be confusion in many jurisdictions over the legal status of
the products of artificial insemination with donor sperm (AID) even
though this technique has been in use for over a century. Kass
(1981:458) contends that it is patently unfair to deliberately deprive children of their natural ties, and that any public policy
which further erodes personal identify is deplorable. For Kass
"clarity about your origins is crucial for self-respect." Similarly,
the President's Commission (1982:65) envisions that these innovations might alter people's sense of family and kinship and increase
the strains on the concept of lineage. Although it is difficult to
speculate on the multitude of legal custody possibilities arising
from sophisticated reproductive techniques, they are bound to be
as significant as are challenges to self-identity and notions of family.

Who ultimately has legal and moral responsibility to care for
the products of technology-mediated procreation? Recent cases involving surrogate mothers (i.e., *In re Baby M*) show how impossible
it is to apply long accepted but now outdated criteria in assigning
responsibility. Who are rightful parents and who decides what is
best for the progeny where the traditional mother-father combination is clouded or no longer appropriate? Recently, adopted children have begun to exercise their right to know their natural parents. What psychological effect might the knowledge that one is the
product of the fertilization of an anonymous donor sperm and
donor egg in a petri dish have on a person? What if one's genetic
roots can be described only as the best of the embryos flushed from
donor women five days after fertilization? Do we want to establish
a society where such information is unimportant to the person or
is it part of human nature to know one's biological roots? To what
extent, if any, is the dignity of human life threatened by the loss of
personal autonomy which derives from one's biological unique-
ness?

Difficulties in defining parental responsibility also are accentuated by the introduction of technologies that allow for prenatal
or genetic intervention. The availability of genetic screening, prenatal diagnosis, and fetal surgery has implications for society's
perceptions of responsible and irresponsible parental behavior. As
the technological ability of the parents to act for the well-being of
the child increases, expansion of the notion of parental responsibil-

ity is certain. Until now, a central tenet of parenting in the United States has been that procreation and parenting represent private and autonomous spheres of personal action. With the permeation of these reproductive intervention techniques, however, the "boundaries of parental responsibility—and hence people's ideas of what it is to be a good parent—may shift rapidly" (President's Commission 1982:65).

On the other hand, should a person or couple who desires only one or two children be denied all the technological help they can muster to produce progeny according to the specifications of their choice? Certainly, it is human to desire that one's children be better off than one's self and that they have all possible advantages. Until recently, these ends could be pursued only through efforts to improve the environment. Now parents have the opportunity to draw upon knowledge and techniques of reproductive research. How far ought they to go in that regard: selective abortion, sex preselection, trait selection, germ plasm marketplaces, artificial or surrogate wombs? More importantly, how far ought we as a society go in encouraging, facilitating, or, perhaps, mandating such decisions?

INCREASING CONSUMER DEMAND FOR HUMAN REPRODUCTION TECHNOLOGIES

The scope of the rapid growth in demand for technology-mediated reproduction will be illustrated in the substantive chapters that follow. Suffice it here to show that this demand presently is considerable and that it will heighten as third-party payers reimburse the costs and commercial enterprises market their products. One reason for the heightened demand is reflected in data on infertility in the United States. Estimates show that somewhere between 8.5 percent (OTA 1988a) and 15 percent (Frankel 1979:93) of all married couples in this country have fertility problems. Some recent estimates have placed the figure even higher. Moreover, the proportion of men and women of childbearing age with fertility problems is increasing throughout the United States (OTA 1988a:4). It is estimated that the sperm count of American males has fallen by over 30 percent in the last half century and that it is continuing to fall. The median count which was estimated to be 90 million sperm per cubic centimeter in 1929, had declined to 60 million in 1979.

Although the causes of this decline are unknown, environmental pollution appears to be a prime suspect. Whatever the cause, nearly 25 percent of all men now have sperm counts so low as to be considered by some researchers to be functionally sterile (Andrews 1981:64).

Similarly, the proportion of women experiencing fertility problems shows dramatic increases. Of the approximately 1.5 million American women who suffer from involuntary sterility, approximately 40 percent are sterile because of diseased fallopian tubes. The highly sensitive oviducts are easily scarred by disease or infection, thus blocking passage of the ovum to the sperm. Scarring can result from pelvic inflammatory diseases or other low-level gynecological infections. Contemporary social patterns, including increased sexual contact of young women with a variety of partners, are linked with increased infertility in women. The epidemic proportions of gonorrhea and, more recently, herpes simplex II and chlamydia among young women promise to accentuate this problem (Schachter and Shafer 1985).

Given these medical circumstances alone, it is not surprising that the demand for reproduction-aiding technologies is escalating. The emergence of these innovations has been met with considerable enthusiasm by couples who desire to have children. Furthermore, several social patterns reinforce the demand for these technologies. First, the availability of healthy newborns for adoption has virtually disappeared in some locales. Among the reasons given for this decline are the development of more effective birth control methods and increased social acceptance of, and education regarding the use and availability of, contraceptives. Widespread use of abortion by unwed women, along with a growing trend of single mothers to keep their babies, have also contributed to this situation. As a result, adoption, once the most common solution to infertility, is no longer a viable option for many couples.

A second social pattern that has created a demand for technology-mediated reproduction is the variety of alternate lifestyles or families that are now commonplace. Lesbian couples who want children without sexual intercourse, and who are most likely unable to adopt, have turned to artificial insemination by donor (AID). Although the number of such couples will remain small, an increasing number of single women might be attracted to technologies that promise them children without the involvement of sex. Also, the high divorce-remarriage rate has resulted in an expansion in the number of men who underwent vasectomies during their first marriage and now desire to have children with their second wife. Although vasectomies can sometimes be reversed, most often the only method of having children is through AID. Similarly, for women who underwent sterilization in their first marriage, in vitro fertilization is frequently the only means of having a child in the second marriage.

Third, the increased availability and attention directed toward these new reproductive technologies appears to be producing a desire on the part of many couples to have their "own" child rather than wait through a long adoption process. This is especially true for older couples who have waited until their careers were established to have children only to find out they are then unable to do so.

Finally, another social pattern which portends increased demand for reproduction technologies is the tendency for many women to postpone parenting until their mid- to late thirties after they have established their careers. Data consistently corroborate that infertility increases with age in both men and women. U.S. data show approximately 8.7 percent infertility among women 25 to 29, 13.6 percent among those aged 30 to 34, 24.6 percent of those 35 to 39, and 27.2 percent of those 40 to 44 (OTA 1988a:4). Although a French study (Schwartz and Mayaux 1982), which found even higher rates of infertility over age 30, sparked considerable debate, including suggestions that women might better postpone careers and concentrate on childbearing in their twenties (DeCherney and Berkowitz, 1982), this pattern is expected to persist. As a result, the demand for technology-mediated reproduction by women who want to start childbearing later in life will intensify. Also, it is critical to note that, as a group, these women are affluent and are likely to be willing to expend substantial resources to have a child.

Together, these various social and technological patterns combine to produce powerful demands for reproduction technologies. Although it is arguable whether these technologies "cure" infertility, for the consumers using them they overcome a disability of substantial consequence. According to Walters and Singer: "Some infertile women may not have a strong desire to have children, and in that case their disability does not trouble them; but others obviously find their disability a major threat to their happiness" (1982:136).

In a survey of couples seen for infertility problems, Freeman and

associates (1985) found that 50 percent of the women and 15 percent of the men reported that infertility was the most stressful
experience of their lives (compared to 13 percent for death and 9
percent for illness or accident). For these couples, the need to have
a child will be manifested by intense demands for such services.
Once the technologies become available and are proven effective,
their diffusion across the country is guaranteed, because the pool
of candidates for technology-mediated procreation is a growing
one.

COMMERCIALIZATION OF REPRODUCTION:
OVERVIEW OF OPTIONS

One of the most disquieting trends in technology-mediated reproduction is the growing commercialization of it. The shift of fertility
research and services from the public sector to the private, profit-
making sector raises serious questions as to what role public institutions ought to take in regulating these businesses. At a deeper
level, clear dilemmas arise in U.S. society regarding commercialization of one of the most personal and revered aspects of our
culture—human reproduction. On the one hand, we highly value
free enterprise and place considerable faith in the marketplace as
an arbiter of supply and demand of goods and services. As noted
earlier, there is a growing demand for a full range of reproduction-
aiding technologies. Why not leave it up to the profit-making sector
to meet these demands much as we do in every other area of human
existence, including health care, which until recently was the bastion of nonprofit public or quasi-public enterprise?

On the other side is the contention that reproduction is special
and that commercializing it somehow degrades it and makes it less
natural and human. Despite our belief in free enterprise, many
persons recoil from the idea of marketing human germ material,
even human embryos, much as we market soap. Moreover, there is
a reaction against the exploitation of the infertility of persons by
an industry formed to turn a profit for its stockholders. This aversion to commercialization of human reproduction is largely emotional, although it has rational components, particularly in the
policy problems it raises for a society that prides itself on maximizing individual autonomy. Despite this hesitancy—and, in some
cases, revulsion—to countenance the emerging enterprises in re-

production, the trend in that direction is unmistakable. A major question is how this trend toward commercialization will affect reproductive choice in the United States. Will it expand procreative rights of individuals, eventually concentrate control of reproduction in the state, or depersonalize reproduction to the extent that it is viewed as just another commercial process? Although these questions are raised throughout this book, several radical future scenarios are presented in order to demonstrate the potential extent of this new revolution in reproduction.

Brave New World of State Control over Human Reproduction

Often alluded to in critiques of human reproductive intervention is Aldous Huxley's *Brave New World*. Published in 1932, Huxley's novel takes place in a society in which human breeding technologies have reached a stage where the state is able to centrally control reproduction. In this society, according to the Director of Hatcheries and Conditioning, social stability, the cornerstone of the state, is perpetuated through a centralized fertilization process. In describing this process to a group of students, he starts with a description of the surgical excision of the ovaries of selected women:

> the operation undergone voluntarily for the good of Society, not to mention the fact that it carries a bonus amounting to six months' salary: continued with some account of the technique for preserving the excised ovary alive and actively developing. . . referred to the liquor in which the detached and ripened eggs were kept; showed them how this liquor was drawn off from the test tubes. . .how the eggs which it contained were inspected for abnormalities, counted and transferred to a porous receptacle; how. . .this receptacle was immersed in a warm bouillon containing free-swimming spermatozoa (and) how the fertilized ova went back to the incubators; where the Alphas and Betas remained until definitely bottled; while the Gammas, Deltas and Epsilons were brought out again, after only thirty-six hours, to undergo Bokanovsky's Process.

The director goes on to exclaim that Bokanovsky's Process, where the egg is subdivided to produce up to ninety-six buds that each develop into "standard men and women; in uniform babies," is one of the "major instruments of social stability."

> For in nature it takes thirty years for two hundred eggs to reach maturity. But our business is to stabilize the population at this mo-

purchasing, at their local medical market, the appropriate pill to guarantee a child of the sex of their choice.

Inherent in this second scenario is the commercial dimension of procreation. Although it would be possible to extend reproductive choice of individuals without dependence on a market system, within the context of the patterns described in this book it is probable that whatever the future brings, commercialized procreation will be a part of it. This, of course, means that the marketplace can be shaped by one of several forces: demands by a consumer public or control by the state. The key to the direction taken seems to depend on the extent to which the state takes an active role in the reproduction of its population.

It is crucial to note here that the major differences in these two scenarios are political and social, not technological. Although there are obvious unique adaptations of technology in each society because of their variant goals and priorities, the levels of sophistication of reproductive technology are similar. The primary disparities between these scenarios are the product of two fundamentally antithetical political ideologies. In the former, reproductive innovations have been developed, introduced, and diffused with the explicit goal of maximizing social stability and efficiency by controlling and institutionalizing human procreation. Contrarily, in the latter, priorities are established on the basis of the extent to which they expand individual procreative choice. Ironically, both scenarios severely challenge traditional conceptions of human reproduction and represent social settings at variance with popular notions of what the future ought to be.

TECHNOLOGY-MEDIATED REPRODUCTION: THREAT OR PROMISE?

In his preface to the second edition of *Brave New World* (1946:xix), Huxley admits that a future where human procreation is a sophisticated manufacturing process under state control is far closer than it had appeared in his original projection of six hundred years: "it seems possible that the horror may be upon us within a single century." Today, it is even more evident that, if we as a society choose that direction, we are capable technologically of reaching a brave new world in considerably less time than Huxley's latter estimate. If a state is determined to mobilize science and technology toward that end, such a goal seems feasible.

Whether or not our society approaches a brave new world is dependent on decisions we make in the very near future, because policies made at this stage are likely to shape succeeding options. Leon Kass (1972) states that "one technical advance makes possible the next and in more than one respect, the first serves as a precedent for the second, the second the third—not just technologically, but also in moral arguments." Our future moral, as well as technical, options are conditioned, and to some extent determined, by how we approach contemporary technological dilemmas. This is most obvious in the area of human reproduction, because of the sequential nature of the techniques. For example, in vitro fertilization opens the way to manipulation of the zygote, to embryo research, and to innumerable other innovations which are possible only after its initial achievement. Decisions made today concerning reproduction technology priorities are especially critical in light of this progressive pattern of development.

Despite the inevitable developmental trends in technology-mediated reproduction and the indications that they could lead to a world where state control of procreation is prominent, at this juncture, American society still has an opportunity to proceed in almost any direction regarding the application of this knowledge. We can establish a context within which individual procreative choice is expanded, or we can move toward a form of social control resembling that of *Brave New World*. It must be reemphasized that although technologies can contribute to either end, ultimately political decisions will dictate the path to be followed.

Plato proposed one of the grandest schemes of selective human breeding 2500 years ago in the *Republic*, where he designed an intricate eugenic program comprising class, as well as age, criteria for selective breeding. "It follows. . .that, if we are to keep our flock at the highest pitch of excellence, there should be as many unions of the best of both sexes, and as few of the inferior as possible, and that only the offspring of the better should be kept."

Although the presence of more sophisticated human breeding techniques might promote the ends of Plato, they are not a sufficient, nor even a necessary, ingredient. David Baltimore (1983:52) sees little about "tinkering with human inheritance" that is "terribly frightening," because in our society we do not accept as appropriate the type of social organization which would be necessary to accomplish the goals of a Plato, a Hitler, or the brave new world. For the President's Commission on the Study of Ethical Problems in Medicine (1982:71), the peculiar social and political circumstances that lead to the attempts to control human reproduction through the coercive power of the state "are not present in this country and are unlikely to occur in the foreseeable future." Contrarily, the inevitable tightening of the economic constraints on health care and social programs is likely to cause tensions between individualistic values and technological applications that intrude upon individual prerogatives in procreation.

This brief discussion of the choices that emerge out of advances in human reproduction technology illustrates the multitude of dilemmas and the intensity of problems we must soon face. On the one hand, there are strong pressures to develop and utilize to the fullest extent these remarkable innovations. Among other things, they hold out the promise of reducing the incidence of many genetic diseases, overcoming infertility of couples who desire children, and providing opportunities for selecting certain characteristics of our progeny. Conversely, because many potential applications of these techniques threaten prevailing values, including the reluctance to interfere with individual reproductive choice, there is fervid opposition to their development and application. Collectively, these technologies require that certain aspects of what it means to be a human be changed. The President's Commission (1982:70) concludes that even the possibility of this alteration "rightly evokes profound concern and burdens everyone with an awesome and inescapable responsibility—either to develop and employ this capability for the good of humanity or to reject it in order to avoid potential undesirable consequences."

The way in which we approach human reproduction in light of the second reproductive revolution is intricately related to what our future society will be. The policy questions regarding regulation of human reproduction, then, are critical to the survival of our society as we know it. We have a very powerful set of technologies, but to date we have not dealt with them realistically. There is an urgent need to face the policy issues raised by reproductive technologies directly and to frame a feasible set of policies that maximizes the benefits and minimizes the dangers to society and its members. The goal of this book is to provide this framework.

CHAPTER TWO

Human Genetic and Reproductive Intervention

AMONG THE most dramatic biomedical technologies are the rapid developments in human genetic and reproductive intervention. Until recently, we had little control over procreation in terms of the genetic "quality" of our progeny. Also, infertile persons had little hope of circumventing their problem. As recently as a generation ago, the capacity to remove fertilization from the secrecy of the womb to the bright lights of the laboratory was inconceivable. Newfound abilities to intervene at the most basic level of the gene are indeed revolutionary. As such, they bring, not only change, but also critical questions as to what implications that change has for individuals and for society as a whole.

Ironically, genetic intervention is controversial especially because of the accelerating succession of advances in knowledge of human genetics and the shortened lead time between basic research and application. Fundamental values tend to change slowly across generations, and so the speed of achievements in genetic technology threatens these values, while allowing little opportunity for careful reflection. As a result, value conflicts are created within a very short time span and soon are elevated to the public policy arena. The tendency of the mass media to oversimplify the technologies and focus on sensational cases often results in exaggerated fears to persons who feel threatened, and unrealistic hope by those who view the technologies as a solution to their problems, thus escalating the debate.

In addition to challenging basic values, human genetics for many persons raises the specter of eugenics and social control. References to a *Brave New World* scenario, in which human reproduction is a sophisticated manufacturing process and a "major instrument for social stability" are commonplace, as are comparisons to Nazi Germany. Moreover, fears of "human genetic engineering," itself often a pejorative expression in this context, are cast in terms of playing God or interfering with evolution. Not surprisingly, opposition to genetic and reproductive intervention in this context is frequently intense.

A complicating factor that heightens opposition to genetic intervention among some groups is the selective nature of genetic diseases. The success of genetic screening efforts often depends upon the ability to isolate high-risk groups. When targeting these groups, however, problems of stigmatization, due process, and invasion of privacy result. The early experience with sickle-cell screening, for instance, led to perceived and real threats to the black community and raised severe criticism of screening efforts. As DNA probes are used to identify individuals at heightened risk for alcoholism, personality disorders, and so forth, the issue of stigmatization is bound to reemerge, thus making any attempts to screen very controversial.

HUMAN REPRODUCTION INTERVENTION

The revolution in human reproduction, which began in the 1960s with the separation of reproduction from sexual intercourse through widespread use of "the pill" and other contraceptive innovations is quickly entering a second phase—one that provides a corollary to the contraceptive revolution by giving us the means to reproduce without sex. Critical public policy issues are now emerging which must be addressed if we are to face the challenges raised by the array of reproductive technologies that alter the givens of human reproduction and allow for many combinations of human germ material outside conventional sexual reproduction.

Technologies of Human Reproduction

Infertility is a growing problem for many American men and women. In 1988, an estimated one in six couples was infertile. Although the causes of infertility are complex and poorly understood, they include environmental, heritable, pathological, and sociobehavioral factors. Even though drug therapy and microsurgical intervention are effective in treating infertility in some instances, couples increasingly are turning to reproductive technologies. According to the OTA (1987:1), the demand for these services is attributable in part to several factors:

1. Couples are delaying childbearing, thereby exposing themselves to the higher infertility rates associated with advancing age.
2. An increased proportion of infertile couples is seeking treatment due to an increased awareness of the availability and successes of modern infertility services, coupled with a decreased supply of infants available for adoption. In 1983, about 50,000 adoptions took place in the United States, but an estimated 2 million couples wanted to adopt.
3. A greater number of physicians offer infertility services than in previous years. An estimated 45,600 physicians provide infertility services, a statistic that exceeds by 25 percent the number of physicians providing obstetric care (1987:1).

The most widely used form of reproduction-aiding technology today is artificial insemination (AI). It is estimated that over 500,000 children in the United States have been born to women fertilized by this method. A major survey estimates that 172,000 women underwent AI in 1986–87, resulting in 35,000 births from AI using husband's sperm and 30,000 from AI utilizing donor sperm (OTA 1988b:3). Although it is the simplest technique, AI still brings physicians and other third parties into the reproductive process. Also, it introduces the concept of collaborative conception. Despite its long history and relatively high use, there are no consistent policy guidelines across the states.

Artificial insemination is a relatively simple medical procedure, although its success depends on a number of technical factors including the quality of the semen specimen and the timing of insemination. Semen obtained by masturbation is deposited by means of a syringe in or near the cervix of the woman's uterus. As the exact timing of ovulation is uncertain, insemination is usually conducted on several consecutive days in order to increase the chance of pregnancy. A success rate of 70 to 80 percent pregnancy, within three to four months of the start of treatment, has been achieved. Although few systematic, long-term studies have been conducted, there is no significant evidence to date of increased mortality or abnormality rates in babies born via AI. Iizuka et al. (1968) conclude that physical and mental development of the AI children is in no way inferior to those in the control group and that in IQ they significantly exceed the control group.

Although the procedures are identical, there are two basic types of AI depending on whether the sperm used is the husband's (AIH) or a donor's (AID—also called donor insemination or DI). While biologically it is irrelevent whether the semen is provided by the husband or a donor, the ethical, psychological, and social problems surrounding AID are more severe. Also, indications for the use of each technique differ. In the past, AIH was limited to the infrequent situation where physical or psychological difficulties precluded fertilization through intercourse. Recently, in combination with the capability to freeze and store sperm, it has become possible to pool several ejaculations from a male with a low sperm count (oligospermia), concentrate them by separating the spermatoza from the semen, and then inseminate the concentration into the wife's cervix.

Artificial insemination with a donor is medically indicated when: the husband is wholly infertile, there is severe RH incompatibility, or the husband is known to suffer from a serious hereditary disorder such as Huntington's disease. Annas (1980:5) notes that although 95 percent of AID practitioners reported that their primary reason for using AID was because of husband infertility, at least 40 percent had used it for other reasons, including 10 percent who had used it to fertilize single women. In addition to its strict clinical uses, AID encompasses a range of possible eugenic applications. By selecting donors according to some predetermined genetic characteristics, AID might be used to promote propagation by means of males with such qualities. Although this positive eugenics approach might benefit human evolution (Muller 1961), there appears to be only limited support for AID to be used for strictly eugenic objectives (Medawar 1969). On the other hand, it has been argued that persons with certain genetic diseases should refrain from propagating (Purdy 1978). Under these conditions, AID could be used as an alternative means of "having children."

AID can be carried out in three ways, each of which contains advantages and disadvantages. The first is through professional services, either at a sperm bank or through an independent physician. Most married couples utilize these services. Some married women and a growing number of single women, however, are utilizing third parties as intermediaries. These liaisons select the donor and arrange the insemination without disclosing the identity of the donor to the woman. A final method of AID is insemination with a donor known by the woman through a direct arrangement between the woman and the donor. In all three cases, the actual insemination might be conducted by a physician or by the woman herself, because the AID procedure is such a simple one, a fact that distinguishes AI from the other reproductive-mediated conceptions discussed later in this book.

AID through a sperm bank or private physician has the advantage of minimizing any risk of future legal suit by the donor for custody or visitation rights. In order to ensure a continuous pool of sperm donors, professional services must guarantee that the donor's identity remain secret. According to Curie-Cohen and associates (1979), in order to guarantee donor anonymity, physicians often keep inadequate records or intentionally inseminate patients with multiple donors in a single cycle. The problem with this approach is that the children of AID have little or no access to medical or genetic records of their biological father's lineage. Nor is there much possibility of the children discovering the identity of their biological father—knowledge which apparently is important for an increasing number of adopted children.

Also, gaining access to professional services is a major problem for some groups, such as single women and lesbian couples. Although Kern and Ridolfi (1982) view this as a violation of these women's fundamental rights to procreate and bear a child under the Fourteenth Amendment, it is unlikely that the courts will actively intervene in the near future to guarantee access, particularly to commercial AID services. This means that third-party arrangements and AID with a known donor might be used by a minority of women. Inceasingly, though, because of the protection afforded by professional services with their accompanying anonymity, most AID will be effectuated through that method.

Although the first reported child who was the product of AID was born a century ago, its use has expanded in the last few decades by the introduction of cryopreservation techniques, which freeze and preserve sperm indefinitely by immersion in liquid nitrogen. Cryopreservation has led to the establishment of commercial sperm banks, some of which now advertise their products to the public. Sperm banks also make it possible for a man to store his semen prior to undergoing a vasectomy as a form of "fertility insurance." More importantly, they also facilitate eugenic programs, such as the Repository for Germinal Choice which inseminates women of "high intelligence" with sperm of "superior men."

In vitro fertilization (IVF) is the procedure by which eggs are removed from a woman's ovaries and fertilized outside her body in a petri dish. The resulting embryos are kept in a culture medium for approximately two days until they reach the four- to eight-cell stage at which point they are transferred (ET) via catheter into the uterus of the women. When successful, the embryos will implant within five days, resulting in a pregnancy. Usually, the retrieval of the mature eggs via laparoscopic surgery is preceded by ovulation induction in which the woman takes a combination of hormones that stimulate her ovaries to "superovulate"—to produce an abnormal number of eggs to be fertilized thus increasing the chances of conception and, ultimately, pregnancy. IVF is indicated when the oviducts are blocked, preventing the egg from passing through the fallopian tubes to be fertilized. One variation of IVF is gamete intrafallopian transfer (GIFT) in which sperm and eggs are transferred directly to the fallopian tubes. Because fertilization takes place in the fallopian tubes instead of a petri dish, GIFT is more acceptable than IVF to some religious groups, such as the Roman Catholic Church. A second variation of IVF is zygote intrafallopian transfer (ZIFT) in which the embryo is placed in the fallopian tube about 18 hours after fertilization.

Andrews (1984:123) estimates that approximately 490,000 American women might be helped by these techniques. The highly sensitive oviducts are easily scarred by disease or infection, which then block passage of the ovum to the sperm. Scarring can result from pelvic inflamatory diseases or other low-level gynecological infections. Contemporary social patterns, including increased sexual contact of young women with a variety of partners, are linked to increased infertility in women. The epidemic proportions of gonorrhea and, more recently, herpes simplex II and chlamydia among young women promise to accentuate this problem (see Sellors et al. 1988:451–456).

In addition to its clinical application to circumvent infertility caused by blocked fallopian tubes, IVF expands considerably the possible combinations of germinal material and further complicates the concept of parenthood. There is no biological reason why the fertilized egg cannot be transferred to a woman other than the one who supplied the egg. IVF, then, enables collaborative conception and the use of surrogate mothers who carry another genetic mother's baby to term. Moreover, there is increasing evidence that the embryo might be transferred to the abdominal cavity of a male, thus enabling male pregnancy. The birth of a baby from a New Zealand woman who had no uterus, and successful male procreation in other species, contribute to the expectation that IVF will soon permit human male pregnancies. One group of transsexual females is already lobbying for such IVF research and applications as part of their desire to "fulfill womanhood in its fullest."

The removal of conception from the secrecy of the womb to under the microscope of the laboratory also enables a wide range of pre-embryo research possibilities (to be discussed in more detail in chapter 3). It will also enable genetic screening, selection, and modification of embryos as these techniques develop. Techniques in which the embryo is physically divided to create twins will permit screening of one embryo—if it "passes the test," its twin can be transferred to the womb for implantation and eventual birth. Cryopreservation of eggs and embryos, in addition to sperm, permits combination of germ materials from persons across generations. Embryo freezing, perhaps combined with twinning, will allow for twins to be born years or even generations apart. Already the ability to freeze embryos has resulted in the birth of nonidentical twins several years apart.

IVF also illustrates the speed at which these technologies become diffused. In 1978, the first IVF baby, Louise Brown, was born in England. In January, 1980, after considerable political debate, Norfolk General Hopsital obtained governmental approval to build the new IVF facility. On December 28, 1981, Elizabeth Carr became the first IVF baby born in the United States. Within eight years, the number of clinics offering IVF expanded to more than 190 and the number of children born through this method is more than 4,000. In response to the rapid growth of IVF clinics, the National IVF/ET Registry was established in 1986. Its first report (Medical Research International 1988) summarized data for 1985 and 1986, collected from the 103 clinics enrolled in the registry.

> There were 2389 and 2864 IVF cycles with embryos transferred in 1985 and 1986, respectively. In 1985 and 1986, 337 (14.1%) and 485 (16.9%) of the transfer cycles, respectively, resulted in clinical pregnancies. The number of cycles with frozen embryos transferred increased from 26 to 112 between 1985 and 1986. In 1986, there were 7 clinical pregnancies through frozen ET. In 1985, there were 56 gamete intrafallopian transfer (GIFT) procedures, whereas in 1986 there were 466 such treatment cycles.

The number of clinical pregnancies by GIFT increased from 3 to 601 between 1985 and 1988, and success rates now average about 30 percent pregnancy for each cycle.

Moreover, most clinics continue to have long waiting lists of women who are willing to pay $4000 to $5000 for a chance to become pregnant. In most cases, the final cost of pregancy is in excess of $25,000, because more than one attempt is necessary. Despite this investment, up to 80 percent of the woman who undergo in vitro fertilization do not become pregnant. Some couples have gone through the process up to eight times without success. Pressures are mounting for insurance companies to cover all or part of the procedure, and some are doing so. In October 1987, Massachusetts became the second state to adopt a statute (following Maryland's 1985 lead) that requires private insurance companies, but not Medicaid, to cover the costs of all treatment designed to overcome infertility, including IVF. If costs are reimbursed in whole or in part by third-party payers, demand will escalate even faster. Once the technologies become available and are proven effective, their diffusion across the country is guaranteed, because the pool of candidates for technology-mediated procreation is a growing one.

Although IVF appears not to cause any danger for the mother, the degree of risk to the developing embryo is still unknown. Based on the very limited data available to date, there is no evidence of an increase in congenital malformations after IVF (Lancaster

1985:861). Major potential sources of damage, however, could be related to development of the ovum (especially if superovulation is employed), the selection of sperm (the female reproductive tract selects against some types of abnormal sperm), the fertilization itself, and the use of freezing techniques to preserve gametes or embryos (Biggers 1981:337). Ironically, while considerable research is needed to test for safety for the embryo, ethical concerns about the research itself preclude adequate human embryo testing.

Embryo lavage, or surrogate embryo transfer (Annas 1984), is an effort to flush embryos from donor women and transfer one or more to the recipient woman. The process entails five major steps:

1. Synchronization of the ovulation times between the donor woman and the recipient woman
2. Insemination of the donor woman with sperm from the infertile recipient's husband
3. Washing out (lavage) the donor's uterus after about five days following fertilization
4. Recovery of the embryo from the lavage fluid
5. Transfer of the embryo to the uterus of the recipient woman

Obviously, sperm could come from a donor rather than the husband of the recipient. The use of multiple donor women is done to maximize the production of an embryo for transfer. Embryo lavage has the advantage of circumventing the need to retrieve eggs through laparoscopy or ultrasound procedures. However, it brings additional parties into the reproductive process and raises serious objections from persons who oppose manipulation of embryos. Also, questions have been raised as to what happens to those embryos that are not transferred to the recipient's uterus. And, though there is no evidence to date based on the very few cases, there is concern that the lavage process might cause harm to the embryo. These issues will become more salient as embryo lavage variations are introduced.

One especially controversial social innovation culminating from these technological breakthroughs is surrogate motherhood. Here an infertile woman and her husband contract with another woman (the surrogate) who agrees to be artificially inseminated with the sperm of the husband. After fertilization, she carries the fetus to term; once the baby is born, she relinquishes her rights to it and gives it to the couple. Surrogate motherhood raises new legal and moral problems because the surrogate must be willing to be inseminated by the sperm of a stranger, carry his baby for nine months, and then give the baby to the couple or the individual man who contracted with her, usually for a fee. The commitment of a surrogate mother is substantial, both physically and emotionally. Moreover, the couple must rely totally on the good faith of the surrogate to keep her promise, because they cannot be assured custody of the child even though the husband is the genetic father.

In addition to these currently used techniques, substantially more revolutionary innovations are forthcoming. Egg fusion, or the combination of the nucleus of one mature egg with that of another, eliminates the need for male genetic material and always produces a female. In an extension of this technique, both eggs could be obtained from the same woman, thus producing a daughter who is totally hers genetically. Another promising technique is micromanipulation of sperm into an egg through zona drilling, which allows for insertion of one selected sperm through the egg's outer membrane (Boldt 1988). In April, 1989, the first baby conceived through micro-insemination sperm transfer (MIST) was born in Singapore (National University Hospital 1989). His conception occurred when sperm from his father (who suffered from an excessively low sperm count) was tranferred via a very fine tube called micro-pipette into an area just outside the egg membrane. Another use of micromanipulation, reported by Rawlins et al. (1988) involves removal of genetic materials from the embryo to correct gross fertilization errors—in this case, an extra male pronucleus.

Reproductive-aiding technologies also overlap with screening and selection technologies. Sperm separation techniques used in conjunction with AID and IVF now provide the means to maximize conception of a child of the desired sex. Increasingly precise genetic diagnosis using molecular probes of embryos prior to transfer will give us the capacity for even greater control over the characteristics of our progeny.

One shared characteristic of all reproduction technologies is that they introduce a third party into what has been a private matter between a man and a woman. The more complex the intervention, the more mediators are necessary. Embryologists, geneticists, and an array of other specialists become the new progenitors. Although the desire of these specialists to help desperate patients may be genuine, their very presence takes control of procreation away from the couple. The willingness of many infertile couples to do (and pay) anything to have a child also encourages commercialization of procreation. The heightened demand raises the potential for exploitation of the consumers of these services. Third-party involvement raises critical questions as to who has access to the technologies. The danger, as in all health care, is a tiered system in which the technologies serve primarily the upper middle class.

Given the trend toward heightened fertility problems of American couples and singles, the demand for these innovations will increase significantly. However, because of their perceived threat to conventional notions of parenthood, family, and procreative autonomy, these technologies are bound to be potentially explosive political issues.

A BRIEF LOOK AT PRENATAL DIAGNOSIS

Although the primary focus of this book is on reproductive mediating technologies, several related sets of innovations are briefly described here because of their intricate relationship with these central innovations. One set of developments involves intervention during the prenatal period. Prenatal technologies permit diagnosis of the health of the fetus and thus allow for increasing parental control over the quality of their progeny. As more sophisticated forms of genetic intervention emerge, the prenatal period will increasingly become a critical time for reproductive choices to be made. The availability of prenatal technologies also raises policy dilemmas similar to those found at the preconceptual stage.

By far the most common technique for detection of genetic disorders in utero is *amniocentesis.* In this procedure, a long thin needle attached to a syringe is inserted through the lower wall of the woman's abdomen and approximately 20 cc of amniotic fluid that surrounds the fetus is withdrawn. This fluid contains some live body cells shed by the fetus (Wertz and Fletcher 1989). These cells are placed in the proper laboratory medium and cultured for approximately three weeks. At this time, karyotyping of the chromosomes is conducted to identify any abnormalities in the chromosomal complement, as well as the sex of the fetus. If indicated, specific biochemical assays can be conducted to identify at least eighty separate metabolic disorders and approximately 90 percent of neural tube defects. If a fetus is prenatally diagnosed as having a severe chromosomal or metabolic disorder, therapeutic abortion is offered to the mother. Although amniocentesis has been conducted as early as the 14th week of pregnancy, some commentators have concluded that waiting until sixteen to eighteen weeks from the beginning of the last menstrual period produces the maximum number of viable cells and optimal safety because of the availability of a greater quantity of amniotic fluid (Golbus et al. 1979).

Amniocentesis is now regarded as a routine clinical procedure, and several successful lawsuits against physicians who failed to advise amniocentesis for patients over 35 have accelerated its use. By 1980, approximately 40,000 women per year were undergoing amniocentesis. Moreover, an article (Adams, Oakley, and Marks 1982:493) in the *Journal of the American Medical Association* on maternal age and births in the 1980s indicated that demand for amniocentesis is bound to increase, because of the trend toward high maternal age in the population. Approximately 85 percent of amniocenteses are conducted for chromosomal evaluation, of which about three-fourths are for women over 35 years of age (Verp and Simpson 1985:22).

The reason for the emphasis on amniocentesis for women over age 35 is that the frequency of chromosomal abnormalities, especially the most common one, Down's Syndrome, increases dramatically with maternal age. Of women having live births in 1980, 29 percent of those aged 35 and older, and 4 percent of younger mothers, underwent amniocentesis (Fuchs and Perreault 1986:77). Previous birth of a child afflicted with Down's Syndrome or other chromosomal abnormality, parental chromosome abnormality, and severe parental anxiety are other reasons for chromosomal evaluation. The remaining 15 percent of prenatal diagnoses are indicated by: (1) previous offspring or close relatives with neural tube defects; (2) the possibility of a sex-linked disorder; or (3) carrier status of both parents for an inborn metabolic disorder, such as Tay-Sachs disease.

Chorionic villus sampling (CVS) is a procedure in which a biopsy is taken from the placenta (which has DNA identical to that of the fetus). Transabdominal CVS extracts a small amount of placental tissue from a needle that is put through the pregnant women's abdomen. Transcervical CVS utilizes a pump-type of sampler to aspirate a specimen of placental tissue under direct visualization of a laparoscope. The advantage of CVS over amniocentesis is that CVS can be conducted as early as the ninth week of pregnancy, thus providing first trimester diagnosis (Elias et al. 1985). The disadvantage of CVS, to date, has been an elevated miscarriage rate. However, according to initial results of an ongoing study conducted by the National Institute of Child Health and Human Development, new CVS techniques are making it just about as safe as amniocentesis for mother and fetus (Goldsmith 1988:3521). If these data are confirmed, because of the ability to conduct CVS much earlier than amniocentesis, CVS will undoubtedly replace it as the preferred approach in the near future. The advantage for the pregnant woman is to give her the same information, but at a time when a much safer abortion is possible, than with the midterm abortions associated with amniocentesis.

A technology that is even more widely used than amniocentesis and that has become indispensable in prenatal diagnosis is *ultrasound*, or "pulse-echo," sonography. This procedure uses high-frequency, non-ionizing, nonelectromagnetic sound waves directed into the abdomen of the pregnant woman to gain an echo-visual image of the fetus, uterus, placenta, and other inner structures. It is a noninvasive technology that is painless for the woman and reduces the need for x-ray scanning procedures. Studies to date have found no harmful long- or short-term hazards to the fetus from diagnostic sonography (Office of Medical Applications of Research 1984). In addition to its use in conjunction with amniocentesis to determine fetal position, fetal age, and amniotic fluid volume, ultrasound can also be used to observe fetal development and movement, as well as to detect some musculoskeletal malformations and major organ disorders (Warsof et al. 1986:33). More sophisticated devices can show images of fetal organs, such as the ventricles and intestines. Ultrasound use is also essential in conjunction with fetoscopy or placental aspiration and in fetal surgery (Quinlan, Cruz, and Huddleston 1986:558).

According to one report, "some authorities believe that all 'high-risk' pregnancies should have at least one sonogram" (Department of Health, Education, and Welfare 1979:39). However, in 1984, a panel of medical and scientific experts, although recognizing the present value of ultrasound in obstetrics and identifying twenty-seven clinical indications where it can be of benefit, advised that "data on clinical efficacy and safety do not allow a recommendation for routine screening at this time" (Office of Medical Applications of Research 1984:672). They further cautioned that ultrasound examinations performed solely to satisfy the family's desire to know the sex of the fetus, to view the fetus, or to obtain a picture of the fetus should be discouraged. Given the broad medical applications of ultrasound, however, its use will continue to escalate. It appears that its fullest development and applications are yet to be realized.

Potentially, a wide variety of hereditary disorders, including hemophilia, and possibly Duchenne muscular dystrophy, not approachable via amniotic samples, might be identifiable through *fetoscopy* (Perry 1985). Fetoscopy is an application of fiber optics technology that allows direct visualization of the fetus in utero. The fetoscope is inserted in an incision through the woman's abdomen, usually under the direction of ultrasound. Although only a very small area of fetal surface can be examined because of current limitation in instrumentation, the fetoscope can be maneuvered around in the uterus to examine the fetus section by section. Fetoscopy is also used to sample fetal blood under direct observation from a fetal vessel on the surface of the placenta. This is accomplished by inserting a small tube into the uterus and aspirating a minute quantity of blood for diagnostic testing. Fetoscopy also has direct therapeutic use in the intrauterine transfusion of fetuses with hemolytic disease and considerable potential for introducing medicines, cell transplants, or genetic materials into fetal tissues in order to treat genetic diseases.

Despite substantial progress in fetoscopy and fetoscopic aspiration in the last decade, they are still considered applied research because of the hazards they pose for the fetus. Escalated rates of prematurity, as well as a miscarriage rate of between 3 and 5 percent, accompany these procedures and must be reduced considerably before fetoscopy can be considered routine medical practice. There is no doubt, however, that fetoscopy is a vanguard technology for future efforts at in utero treatment of genetic disease and for fetal surgery.

Approximately 6000 infants are born each year in the United States with neural tube defects, the majority equally divided between anencephaly and spina bifida (Main and Mennuti 1986:1). Although there is a 2 to 3 percent risk that the defect will recur after one affected pregnancy, over 90 percent of neural tube defects occur without prior indication that prenatal testing is warranted (Macri and Weiss 1982:633). In 1973, however, an association between elevated levels of maternal serum alpha-fetoprotein (AFP) and open neural tube defects was reported. Since then, research on screening has proliferated.

The level of AFP is determined from either amniotic fluid or maternal serum collected between the fourteenth and twentieth week of pregnancy. At present, approximately 90 percent of neural tube defects can be diagnosed through use of these tests. Because dynamic changes in AFP levels occur normally during this period of gestation, more critical control data and more advanced techniques for quantification are required. Also, since there is some overlap in the distribution of AFP levels in amniotic fluid and maternal serum both in pregnancies with neural tube defects and in normal pregnancies, there is still a false positive rate in approximately 1 in 10,000 cases.

Although measurement of AFP in amniotic fluid samples taken from women at known risk for fetal neural tube defects is recommended, mass serum AFP screening from unselected pregnant women is regarded as premature. The recent approval by the FDA of diagnostic kits to test for neural tube defects spurred controversy by consumer groups and scientists alike. Primary objections focused on the high rate of false positives, the gross nature of the test, and the possibility that women would abort fetuses solely on the basis of this preliminary screening device, when the actual probability of having an affected child is very low. The AMA Council on Scientific Affairs (1982:1478) emphasized the need for "intensive statewide pilot" projects to discover the appropriateness and efficacy of screening in the United States. In contrast, Main and Mennuti (1986:16) recently concluded that "voluntary maternal serum screening should be offered to the general obstetric population in the United States." Another observer (Simpson 1986:202) cautions, however, that such screening must be coupled with ultrasound examination and is suitable only for certain parents. It appears that use of both maternal serum AFP screening and amniocentesis to identify neural tube defects will become more common in the near future.

These techniques give us the ability to reduce the incidence of genetic disease, but at this time they do so primarily by eliminating the affected fetus (through selective abortion), not treating the disease. Future developments in gene therapy might shift emphasis toward treatment, but prenatal diagnosis will continue largely to expand parental choice only to the extent that it allows them to terminate pregnancies of affected fetuses. Thus, it will continue to be a policy issue congruent with abortion.

Another policy dilemma centers on who makes the decision to use the technologies, because anything that can be done voluntarily might also be coerced. If prenatal diagnosis were to become legally mandated by imposing tort liability on those persons whose failure to use it resulted in harm to the fetus, then its very availability could limit the freedom of women who chose not to use it. What if, after a physician recommends that a woman at high risk for a Down's Syndrome infant have amniocentesis, she refuses, and has a child with that chromosomal abnormality? Will she be legally liable for the wrongful life of the defective infant? Will her action be seen by the community as irresponsible? What if she undergoes amniocentesis, finds out that the fetus is affected, but refuses because of religious objections, to abort the fetus?

HUMAN GENETIC TECHNOLOGY

The precursor issues in human genetic intervention have arisen from carrier screening techniques. The primary clinical objective of screening for carrier status is to identify those individuals who, if mated with another person with that same particular genetic trait, have a 25 percent chance of having offspring with the disease. Once identified, parents with carrier status can be offered prenatal diagnosis, if it is available for that disease, or at least be educated as to the risk that they take in having children. Because the carriers do not have a disease, genetic screening of this type is indirect. It benefits not the health of those screened but rather the potential persons who have a one-in-four chance of having the disease if they are conceived and born.

Carrier screening programs have been in effect for almost two decades in many states and localities for Tay-Sachs disease and sickle-cell anemia. The sickle-cell programs have been especially controversial because the trait is concentrated in the black population and, unlike Tay-Sachs screening which has always been voluntary, sickle-cell screening started out as mandatory in many states. Carrier screening tests for many recessive genetic diseases and even more precise genetic trait markings will be available in the near future. The most rapid developments have been in the area of DNA probes to identify polymorphisms (genetic variations) that mark a particular trait. Following the discovery of such a molecular probe for the Huntington's disease gene in 1983, efforts have been initiated to identify genetic markers for Alzheimer's disease (Kolata 1986c), manic depression (Kolata 1986a), malignant melanoma (Kolata 1986d), schizophrenia (Barnes 1988), cystic fibrosis (Roberts 1988), and a host of other conditions. The identification of the retinoblastoma gene on chromosome 13 and the discovery of its linkage to breast cancer have led to considerable excitement over the genetic bases of cancer (Marx 1988). In addition, considerable attention is being directed toward genetic factors that might predispose a person to alcohol abuse.

A major research initiative is underway to map the entire human genome, i.e., to identify the placement of all the genes on all the chromosomes (Lewin 1987). One particularly sensitive area of research is directed toward discovering which genes are associated with intelligence. Work on the "fragile-X" chromosome is the first wave (Partington 1986). Eventually, genetic tests will allow scientists to identify not only the course of genetic abnormalities, but also traits that put certain individuals at higher risk for susceptibility to a host of environmental factors. Nolen and Swenson (1988) term these less determinative genes "contingency genes" since they may cause a disease, but only if unknown genetic and environmental factors conspire.

Ironically, these new capabilities accentuate, rather than reduce, the political/legal/ethical issues of genetic counseling and screening. When screening leads to aversion or treatment of genetic disease, the issues, though often controversial, are reasonably straightforward. However, when screening involves identifying heightened risk or susceptibility for particular conditions, it is considerably more problematic. When it is based on controversial assumptions, such as recent media stories on research involving the possible tie between height and I.Q., it is politically explosive. As new diagnostic tests and genetic probes emerge, public expectations will intensify and the demand for accessibility to information derived from such efforts heighten. Once the tests become accepted as legitimate by policy makers, it is likely that legislatures and courts will recognize professional standards of care that incorporate them. Recent legislation in California that requires physicians to inform pregnant patients of the availability of alpha-fetoprotein tests (Steinbrook 1986), and similar court pressure involving a variety of prenatal tests, attest to the public policy dimensions inherent in these applications.

Additional public policy dilemmas emerge in genetic screening as more precise and inclusive tests give us the capacity to screen out people because they are at high risk for a disease or condition.

Increasingly, genetic counselors will face pressures from employers and insurance companies for access to information obtained from these tests (Kolata 1986b). This is not a new issue but one which has been building for the last several decades in conjunction with sickle-cell carrier screening and occupational workplace screening (Hubbard and Henifin 1985). Holden (1982:336) points out that although there are "probably thousands of genetic deficiencies that render individuals unusually vulnerable to certain chemicals," only a few presently are known. To date the most commonly screened traits have been the sickle-cell trait; glucose-6-phosphate dehydrogenase deficiency (G6PD), which can predispose carriers to a hemolytic crisis causing anemia from exposure to certain chemicals such as naphthalene; and alpha-1 antitrypsin (AAT), which can predispose individuals to lung disorders and emphysema from exposure to lung irritants.

There are at least three potential approaches to workplace genetic screening. First, voluntary genetic testing at the worksite could be provided by the employer to provide the individual employee with health risk information. As long as confidentiality of the results are ensured and have no bearing on the employee's status, such testing poses no severe policy problems. Second, mandatory prehiring testing to exclude susceptible workers from environments hazardous to their health could be instituted. Unlike the voluntary tests, because this screening involves discrimination based on genetic status, it raises critical policy questions. However, if the result leads to protection of the employee's health by minimizing a risk uncovered by the tests, it might pass constitutional scrutiny. The third approach to genetic screening in the workplace might follow discovery of DNA markers for genetic susceptibility to such conditions as alcoholism, heart disease, diabetes, and mental illness. If employers require such tests as a precondition to employment and refuse to hire those persons who are identified as bearing such a risk, a new category of discrimination has emerged.

Many employers feel they should have access to data showing that an employee is at heightened risk for occupational hazards, and some companies have initiated their own genetic screening programs, with considerable controversy (Matthewman 1985). Although usually defended on the grounds that it is done for the employee's benefit, such action also reflects a fear of potential liability suits, either from the employee at a later time or from others who might be harmed by the actions of that employee. The potential for DNA probes to identify persons at risk for alcoholism, Alzheimer's disease, manic depression, and so forth accentuate the issue of how much information should be given employers. When, if ever, is the patient's right to privacy to be sacrificed for the interests of the employer? Under what circumstances does the genetic counselor's responsibility to society outweigh his or her responsibility to the patient? As more knowledge is gained about specific susceptibilities related to genetic traits and more accurate tests are found for a wide variety of these traits, debate on workplace screening will heighten. Harsanyi and Hutton (1981:248) expect that the "art of prediction" of screening genetic markers "will be refined to the point where an individual's identification with various groups, along with the genes that he carries, will pinpoint the risks he faces from specific environmental conditions." They go on to contend (262) that, although the workplace should be made as safe as possible for all workers, those who are found to be at greater risk should "either find another job or accept responsibility for the illness to which they are predisposed."

Insurance companies, too, have a substantial stake in data obtained through these methods. Life insurance companies, which traditionally have excluded people who are poor health risks, surely are interested in the results of tests which place certain individuals at high risk for any of the conditions or diseases outlined here. Likewise, health insurance companies, particularly in light of recent developments in such competitive models as health maintenance organizations (HMOs), will want access to test results, particularly if the tests are funded by third-party payments. Insurers know that a large proportion of health care costs are attributable to a small proportion of their members. If tests are available to identify individuals who are genetically predisposed to ill health or to such conditions as alcoholism which increase health care costs, third-party carriers will be under severe economic pressure to identify those persons and eliminate coverage for them, thus reducing overall costs substantially. As with employers, genetic counselors are bound to be at the center of these competing pressures for information on the results of genetic tests.

Although the courts have upheld the constitutionality of premarital tests in instances of communicable diseases, screening for genetic traits certainly is more problematic from a public health rationale. Given the current state of genetic technology, premarital screening would focus on testing the prospective husband and wife for carrier status, presumably for recessive diseases such as sickle-cell anemia, galactosemia, or Tay-Sachs disease. Such a program would be effective only if couples so identified altered their reproductive plans either by not procreating or by making full use of available prenatal diagnostic technologies. It is not clear how such a program would be enforced once the couple had been informed of their "genetic status." At present, there is considerable disagreement about the need for, or effectiveness of, carrier screening as a precondition to marriage (Blank 1981:129).

HUMAN GENE THERAPY

It is foreseeable that the development of techniques to diagnose genetic disorders will lead to some capacity to provide gene therapy. Although extensive human gene therapy is not imminent, at least six major research centers in the United States are working to develop techniques that will permit such treatment (Marx 1986). These techniques would correct genetic defects, not by environmental manipulation but, instead, by acting directly on the DNA in the affected person's cells. One approach, which has been tried on some victims of thalassemia and sickle-cell anemia, might be to switch on certain genes which would otherwise be inactive, so that they can take over the job of the defective genes. Another possible approach, gene therapy, involves the introduction of normal genes into chromosomes of cells that contain defective genes in the hope that the manipulated cells will ultimately replace the defective ones, thus curing the patient (Selden et al. 1987).

The research emphasis today is on somatic cell therapy—where genes are inserted into particular body cells other than the germ cells (sperm, egg, and cells that give rise to them). Because somatic cell gene therapy does not affect the germ line, the genes conveyed through the procedure will not appear in the recipient's progeny. A type of gene therapy considerably more controversial than replacement of a defective gene in somatic cells is the intervention in germline cells—those which contribute to the genetic heritage of offspring.

> In this case, gene therapy has the potential to affect not only the individual undergoing the treatment but his or her progeny as well. Germline gene therapy would change the genetic pool of the entire human species, and future generations would have to live with that change, for better or worse (Olson 1986:50).

Technical difficulties, in combination with ethical concerns, make it extremely unlikely that germline gene therapy will be attempted in the near future, even though theoretically it is the most effective means of therapy. According to Selden et al. (1987:1071):

> From an ethical perspective, modifying the germ line would change, at best slightly, subsequent generations of humans, and the long-term effects would not be entirely predictable. From a practical perspective, germ-line transfer is relatively inefficient; the fate of the injected genes cannot be predicted, and perhaps most important, with few exceptions it would be impossible to determine the future phenotype of a single cell or early-cleavage embryo.

According to W. French Anderson (1984) of the National Heart, Lung, and Blood Institute, the first diseases selected for treatment with somatic cell gene therapy will share several characteristics. First, they will arise from a defect in a single gene that causes the loss of an enzyme—a loss with potentially lethal consequences, severe suffering, and premature death. To date, only a few of the more than 200 single genes known to cause human disorders have been isolated and reproduced through genetic engineering so their copies can be inserted into cells. Second, these diseases will be treatable through genetic manipulation of bone marrow cells, because techniques have been developed to remove these cells from the body, transform them with recombinant DNA, and reintroduce them into the body. Although it might be possible in the future to genetically manipulate skin cells or even tissues and whole organs, to date bone marrow cells are the only cells conducive to this kind of treatment (Olson 1986:45). Finally, the genes responsible for the diseases must have a fairly simple kind of regulation—preferably an "always-on" type.

This move from the diagnostic to the therapeutic ends of genetic intervention reiterates many policy issues regarding the role the government ought to play in encouraging or discouraging research and application of such intervention. This move also raises ethical questions concerning parental responsibilities to their children, societal perceptions of children, the distribution of social benefits, and our definition of what it means to be a human being.

Despite these concerns, there is a growing consensus among persons who have studied somatic gene therapy that it would be unethical to deny this treatment to desperately ill patients once the basic technical conditions of delivery, expression, and safety are satisfied (Olson 1986:48). Somatic cell gene therapy under these conditions differs little in its practical application from traditional treatments, particularly bone marrow and organ transplantation. The only difference is that this therapy operates at the gene level. Grobstein and Flower (1984:14), however, suggest that if reproductive health includes the probability of having genetically normal offspring, that individual could claim an ethical right not to be deprived of germline repair since, without it, all offspring would at least be carriers of the gene. "Although somatic cell therapy might be provided in each generation, the argument to rid the lineage of the defective genes once and for all might prove compelling."

SEX PRESELECTION TECHNOLOGIES

Interest in sex selection is certainly not new. According to Hughes (1981), infanticide has long been practiced in many cultures in order to choose sex. According to the Office of Technology Assessment (1981:312), current interest in sex selection stems from animal research where the financial benefits could be high if, for instance, the sex of the progeny of dairy cattle could be predetermined. Public demand, however, has shortened considerably the lag time between animal and human application of these techniques. Although estimates vary as to when sex preselection will become widely available for humans, sex selection kits have already been marketed in the United States by Pro-Care Industries, Ltd., under the name Gender Choice. These "child selection kits" sold for $49.95 and contained directions, thermometers, and paraphernalia for monitoring vaginal mucus. The kits, available in pick and in blue, were withdrawn in 1987 when the FDA declared that some of the implied claims on the packages and advertisements had not been substantiated (Hrdy 1988:64).

The approaches which appear to offer the best chances of success in human application at present are based on the fact that each sperm cell carries either an X chromosome or a Y chromosome and that sex of the progeny is determined by which type of sperm fertilizes the egg. The goal of sex preselection is to control which type of sperm fertilizes a particular egg. To aid in reaching this objective, some recently discovered characteristics of these two types of sperm are invaluable. First, in any male ejaculation there are more Y-bearing sperm than X-bearing sperm. In addition to being more numerous, Y-bearing sperm are smaller, less dense, and move faster than their X-bearing counterparts. Conversely, the

Y-bearing sperm die sooner and are more readily slowed down by normal acidic secretions of the vagina. However, they are less inhibited than the X-bearing sperm by the alkaline environment of the uterus, once past the vagina.

Within the context of this new knowledge about the sperm, most current research on sex preselection is aimed at developing accurate and reliable sperm separation techniques. Techniques currently being used to do this include various sedimentation processes, centrifugation, and electrophoresis. Once the desired sperm concentrations are isolated, they are inseminated into the recipient woman's uterus by artificial insemination techniques. Gametrics, Ltd., has franchised an albumin density gradient method patented by Ronald Ericsson, which is based on the assumption that Y-bearing sperm swim faster than X-bearing. Gametrics, Ltd. reports that its franchised centers have a success rate of 86 percent for male selection and 74 percent for female selection, although Carson (1988:17) disputes those figures.

Another possible means of separating the X- and Y-bearing sperm is to insert a special type of diaphragm in the woman's reproductive tract to screen out the larger X-bearing sperm and allow passage to the egg of male sperm only. While Lieberman (1968:27) contends that this technique holds considerable promise for widespread use in humans, Hartley and Pietraczyk (1979:234) point out that because sperm are microscopic in size, designing such a membrane presents a yet unsolved technical difficulty. Other promising sex preselection techniques include the use of special foams or jellies developed to affect the motility of one or the other type of sperm. These could also be used in combination with the special diaphragm or, perhaps, with prophylactics designed to screen out the X-bearing or Y-bearing sperm. Although we appear far from translating sex preselection technology into acceptable, simple, and usable methods of application, sex selection is now within the grasp of human endeavor. Moreover, when analyzed within the framework of the frantic research activity in other areas of genetic and reproductive intervention, it seems obvious than control of human characteristics other than sex is within the horizon.

Policy Issues in Sex Preselection

As American couples have fewer children, there is strong evidence that they are willing to use technologies that offer control over the characteristics of their progeny. Although preference for a child of a particular gender is less clear in the United States than in many other cultures, survey data since the 1960s do indicate a preference for a son as the first child born and a daughter as second (Veit and Jewelewicz 1988:939). However, the availability of sex preselection techniques (as opposed to the use of amniocentesis/abortion for terminating the undesired fetus) combined with the trend toward one- and two-child families undoubtedly will produce a broad demand. As sex preselection techniques move from the highly intrusive to less intrusive methods, demand will increase. The establishment of for-profit sex selection services will develop to meet this demand because it is unlikely that existing nonprofit fertility clinics will be able to make a commitment to these non-medically indicated methods, except in those few instances where it is indicated to avert sex-related genetic diseases. Part of the controversy over the development and diffusion of sex preselection innovations centers on attitude data that suggest that males would more often be selected for, especially where couples desire only one child, if safe, effective, and inexpensive techniques were widely available.

Although the scope of sex preselection applications in the United States is unclear at present and no simple, reliable and usable method enjoys wide acceptance by the research community, demand for services is accelerating as fragmented reports of success are covered by the mass media. Unlike in vitro fertilization and other techniques discussed here, the potential market for a reliable and less intrusive method is not limited to a small portion of the public. It also seems to be an area where latent desires of many persons to control the gender of their progeny could be exploited by an industry that markets sex selection products and services. It takes little imagination to picture an advertising campaign designed to market these services to a public that embraces technologies promising to satisfy deep-seated goals.

At least seventy clinics in the United States currently are using variations of the sperm separation procedure to select sex-specific sperm. Although most clinics are primarily experienced in choosing Y-bearing or male-producing sperm, several are working with both sex chromosomes. In 1984 researchers at Swedish Hospital in Seattle claimed a 96 percent accuracy rate in isolating X-bearing sperm by using a sperm sifting process. Their procedure utilizes a three-foot-long, pencil-thin glass column filled with a gel. The semen filters down through the gel and drains into a series of test tubes. Researchers pick the three to five tubes with the cloudiest material and sample each. They stain each sample with a yellow fluorescent dye and examine all of them by microscope under mercury vapor light. Male chromosomes show up with a bright yellow spot while female ones do not show up at all. The sperm sample with the highest concentration of X-bearing sperm is artificially inseminated into the women.

Although Swedish Hospital inseminates the woman the same day as the sperm separation procedure is conducted, there is no biological reason why cryopreservation could not be used to store the sperm sample for future insemination. When refined, techniques such as this one could be routinely used in combination with AID or in vitro programs to maximize the chances of producing a child of the desired sex. A 1988 survey found that 14 percent of AID practioners regularly offer sperm separation for preconception sex selection (OTA 1988b:41). In addition to overcoming infertility problems, this procedure would also allow the couple an opportunity to select the sex of their progeny with a high degree of accuracy. In a competitive market, the addition of sex selection might be an attractive one for some couples, despite the ethical problems it raises concerning the manipulation of the reproductive process.

STERILIZATION

Ironically, one of the most persistent social policy issues in human reproduction is the converse of the reproduction-mediating technologies, sterilization. Moreover, new technological developments in human sterilization promise to complicate rather than to resolve the constellation of constitutional, political, and social problems surrounding the termination of fertility. Most prominent among this array of emerging techniques are efforts at reversible sterilization methods that are less intrusive than traditional surgical techniques.

The interest in reversible sterilization can be understood best by examination of the convergence of several social and technical patterns. First, voluntary sterilization has become a popular method of birth control, the only truly effective method. Studies of contraception practices demonstrate a clear and definite trend toward increased use of sterilization for birth control. A recent survey by

Forrest and Henshaw (1983) found that American women who practice birth control rely most often on sterilization of themselves or their male partners. The data imply that 11.6 million couples depend on sterilization while some 9.9 million women use birth control pills. Over 17 million persons in the U.S. have been sterilized; worldwide, sterilization is by far the single most used form of fertility control.

Long-term fertility control is as elusive now as it was two decades ago. Most couples still elect to have small families while they are young; they are then faced with up to twenty years of fertility control after completion of their family. Rather than using a form of contraception which is at best inconvenient and not fully effective and is at worst a significant hazard to the woman's health, more couples are opting for sterilization as a permanent contraception solution.

A complicating factor that produces an increased demand in the United States for reversible methods is the extremely high divorce-remarriage rate of the 1970s and 1980s. Individuals who were sterilized voluntarily and enthusiastically during their first marriage remarry and decide that their sterilized state is unacceptable under the changed marital circumstances. Renewed interest in childbearing with their new partners often results in attempts to have sterilization reversed. Also, some women who had voluntarily undergone sterilization for personal reasons (e.g., career, job security, desire not to have a family) are deciding later in life that they want a family. Whatever the motivation, there is a salient and accelerating demand for reversal by both men and women. Although most individuals choosing sterilization are reasonably certain they wish to terminate their fertility permanently, a growing number are demanding a form of safety net in case of unforeseen situational changes.

Despite considerable strides in the technology for reversing "permanent" sterilization procedures, the Association for Voluntary Surgical Contraception still considers it standard procedure to advise women undergoing tubal sterilization and men undergoing vasectomy that these are permanent methods of fertility control which may be reversible. Even when a highly trained surgeon uses the most refined instruments and newest techniques, the chances for reversal of tubal ligations and vasectomies may not be high. In addition, some sterilization techniques destroy major sections of the fallopian tubes or vas deferens and make reversal virtually impossible. Current research, therefore, emphasizes techniques designed to be reversible from the start.

Reversible Sterilization Techniques

Of the many current research approaches, the technique that may drastically revise concepts of sterilization and contraception is the removable silicone plug (RSP). This method involves the occlusion of the fallopian tubes with flexible silicone plugs. Unlike conventional sterilization procedures, RSPs are specifically designed to be removed at a later date, to "reverse" the procedure and permit childbearing (Wimberly 1982:1).

This procedure makes use of developments in fiber optics so that the physician can observe the installation of the silicone in the fallopian tubes. A hysteroscope is introduced through the cervix and into the uterine cavity. A liquid silicone mixture is pumped into the oviduct where it solidifies in approximately five minutes. A nylon retrieval loop placed in the silicone allows for removal of the plug by grasping the loop with a forceps and literally "pulling the plug."

The RSP procedure takes less than one hour in an out-patient surgical facility and several follow-up sessions. Reversal is expected to be a relatively simple office procedure, although the clinical testing thus far has focused only on the implantation. Clinical trials conducted in the early 1980s demonstrated success rates in occluding the fallopian tubes of between 80 and 90 percent. Removable silicone plugs are currently being offered as a sterilization technique in many clinics, although the consent form to be signed by the patient usually describes it as a technique that might be reversible—no guarantees. Despite cautions that questions of reversibility are yet unanswered (Wimberley 1982), RSP shows great promise and thereby challenges currently held notions of sterilization as always irreversible (Cooper and Houck 1983:268). Initial successes will stimulate increased demand for reversal services. It is not too early for third-party payers to investigate the potential demand for and costs of providing these services.

In addition to RSPs, various other approaches have been proposed to block the passage of the egg from the ovaries through the fallopian tube. Trials are now proceeding with many of these methods, including fimbrial prosthesis, hug plastic clips, tubal hoods,

Teflon plugs, and a variety of innovative procedures involving burying the fimbrial end of the fallopian tubes. Although theoretically these procedures may be more reversible, according to Henry (1980:c107), "there is no information available to date either on reversals performed or on subsequent pregnancy rates."

Although most research on reversible sterilization techniques to date has been directed at the fallopian tubes, a vas deferens occlusion device has been developed and tested in primates (Zaneveld et al. 1988). The device consists of two silicone plugs held together with a nylon suture. Implantation of the plugs is done by making two small puncture holes in the vas deferens and inserting the plugs. Upon device removal in two primate studies, all subjects ejaculated sperm again at normal concentrations and motility. According to Zaneveld et al. (1988:527), these preliminary results indicate the potential contraceptive use of the device and encourage its validation in men. The simplicity of the device, its effectiveness, and its reversibility should make it a procedure of preference for men who are considering undergoing vascectomy.

Contraceptive Implants

The search for a long-term, reversible method of fertility control has also led to expanding research into subdermal hormonal implants. These implants provide programmed medication that meters the steroid into the surrounding tissue and maintains the blood level in the desired range. The rods or capsules containing the contraceptive steroid are surgically implanted and have expected effectiveness from one to seven years.

The most extensively tested version, NORPLANT, was developed by the Population Council and is manufactured in Finland. It has been tested on over 16,000 women worldwide (Affandi et al. 1987). NORPLANT consists of six silicone rubber capsules, each about the size of a match. The capsules are filled with synthetic progestin, which suppresses ovulation and causes a thickened cervical mucus which inhibits sperm penetration. Under a local anesthetic, the capsules are surgically implanted under the skin of the upper arm in a fanlike fashion. This procedure takes approximately ten minutes and leaves no visible signs. Because the progestin is time-released at low doses, it reduces the risk of overdosing associated with self-administered methods of contraception. The low daily dosage, in addition to the absence of estrogen, is expected to reduce substantially the risks of strokes and blood clots associated with some forms of birth control pills.

NORPLANT, which provides contraceptive protection for five or six years or until the capsules are removed, is welcomed by family planning clinics which have problems of education and compliance in using techniques which require self-administered daily mainte-nance. For individual women, NORPLANT and other subdermal implants will serve as a convenient and, perhaps, safer alternative to the pill. This option will also most likely reduce the number of tubal ligations performed in the United States.

One problem with NORPLANT is that the capsules are nonbiod-egradable and must therefore be surgically removed upon expira-tion. Clinical trials for biodegradable systems that eliminate the need for removal are now underway, although they are not as far along as NORPLANT. One such system, now being researched at the National Institutes of Health, is a polymer implant that also delivers time-released progestin. As it expires after five or so years, however, it vanishes, thus eliminating the need for surgical re-moval. Whatever system becomes the method of choice, in combi-nation with reversible sterilization techniques, contraceptive im-plants promise to revolutionize fertility control. As discussed in chapter 6, however, their very availability raises critical policy issues as well.

POLICY ISSUES IN REPRODUCTIVE TECHNOLOGY

At the very least, these rapid advances in reproductive technology force us to reevaluate our beliefs concerning reproduction and the right of procreation. In a broader sense, they challenge traditional notions of parenthood. Now we must learn to distinguish among the genetic parents (who contribute the germ material), the biolog-ical mother (who carries the fetus to term), and the legal parents, one or both of whom might also be the genetic parents. Moreover, the extent to which these "artificial" methods of reproduction in-volve considerably more individuals (often third parties with a commercial interest) than the "natural" method means that pro-creation is no longer a private matter between a man and a woman. One of the dilemmas raised by these technologies is that, depend-ing upon their specific application, they can be viewed as either extending procreative rights or constraining those same rights. Every reproductive technology has a variety of clinical and eugenic applications, depending upon the motivation of the persons using it.

No issue in the last decades has been more controversial among the American public than that of reproductive choice. The right to privacy in reproduction has been at the center of the women's movement for equal status in a society where the prime role of women in reproduction often has been used to deny them equality. The progression of Supreme Court decisions on procreative privacy beginning with *Skinner v. Oklahoma*, continuing with *Griswold v. Connecticut* and *Eisenstadt v Baird*, culminating in *Roe v. Wade*, and reiterated by *City of Akron v. Akron Center for Reproductive Health* and *Thornburgh v. American College of Obstetricians and Gynecologists* has clearly enunciated a constitutional right of a woman not to conceive or bear a child if she so desires and thus have access to contraception, sterilization, and abortion without state interference. In the 1986 *Thornburgh* ruling, for instance, the Court invalidated six provisions of the Pennsylvania Abortion Control Act which were viewed as interfering unduly with the woman's privacy. Despite significant violation of this right in practice, as a concept, the right to reproductive privacy is well established. However, given recent shifts in the Court balance—and their ruling (*Webster v. Reproductive Health Services*) in July 1989 that upheld a Missouri statute that affirms that human life begins at conception and prohibits the use of public funds, employees, and facilites for abortion-related services not necessary to save the life of the mother— there is growing fear by prochoice advocates of a regression of abortion rights.

Although abortion continues to be a volatile issue, the complementary issue of whether all women (and men) have a corresponding right to have children is more problematic. If there is a right to have children, are there any limits that can be imposed as to the number or "quality" of those progeny? For instance, is there a duty of carriers of genetic disease to refrain from having children from their own germ material and utilize "collaborative conception" technologies such as AID or embryo transfer? Does a woman have a responsibility to avail herself of prenatal diagnostic techniques to identify "defective" fetuses and either abort or, if possible, treat the fetus? At least thirteen women have been ordered by courts to undergo caesarean sections against their wishes, for the benefit of the fetus (Blank 1986:464ff). Should they, as a matter of public policy, also be required to have their body invaded to permit surgery on the fetus in utero? If so, who makes the policy and how is it implemented?

Until now, reproductive choice largely has been framed as a negative right which assures only that the choice can not be constrained without a "compelling state interest." In the absence of a state interest that overrides the choice of the individual, she or he has a right to reproduce as long as the action does not harm a constitutionally defined person. The emergence of reproductive and genetic technologies drastically extends the potential scope of procreative choice, but ironically also threatens the rights to privacy in reproduction that have been gained by women in the last two decades.

Reproduction technologies raise the logical extension of reproductive autonomy as a positive right—a claim upon society to guarantee, through whatever means possible, the capacity to reproduce. If the right to procreation is interpreted as a positive one, then an infertile person might have a constitutional claim to these technologies. Under such circumstances, individuals who are unable to afford those treatments necessary to achieve reproductive capacity could expect society to guarantee access. A woman with blocked fallopian tubes would have a claim to corrective surgery or in vitro fertilization. An infertile man would be ensured access to artificial insemination or corrective surgery, if that is possible. Once procreative rights are stated as positive, however, drawing reasonable boundaries becomes difficult. Does a woman who is unable to carry a fetus to term because of the absence of a uterus or a high-risk condition have a legitimate claim on a surrogate mother who would do so? Wherever the lines are drawn, some individuals are likely to have limited opportunity to have children. The advent of the new technologies of reproduction raises serious questions for procreative choice. Any shifts toward a positive-rights perspective will accentuate the already growing demand for these technologies, encourage entrepreneurs to provide a broad variety of these reproductive services, and, most importantly, put increasing pressures on the government to fund these services.

The new knowledge regarding the transmission of genetic disease, along with the capability to identify carriers of a growing number of deleterious traits, raises another question. Do carriers of recessive genes and persons with dominant diseases have a duty to refrain from procreating? or, if not, to utilize collaborative conception technologies such as artificial insemination or embryo transfer so that these deleterious genes are not transmitted to their offspring? (See chapter 4 for a detailed discussion.)

With current techniques in artificial insemination, cryopreservation, and embryo transfer, these individuals no longer need refrain from conception in order to protect their offspring. Now, for instance, if a husband is suspected of carrying a dominant gene for Huntington's disease, he can use the services of a sperm bank. Although this process eliminates his biological contribution to the child, it also eliminates the 50 percent risk of the child's having the disease. Similarly, if both persons in a couple are identified as carriers of a recessive disease they can: (1) take a 25 percent chance that a child will have the disease and live with it; (2) undergo prenatal diagnosis if available for that disease and abort the fetus if it is identified as having the disease; or, (3) use reproductive technology, such as artificial insemination, and be content with a healthy child, albeit one which is not genetically their own.

Although these options are currently open to couples, the key quesiton is whether a couple has the responsibility to undertake options two or three and, thereby reduce the chance of bearing a child with an avertable genetic disease? Does the child born with a genetic disease have a cause of action against a physician who fails to advise the use of artificial insemination in a case of a disease that cannot be diagnosed prenatally? If the physician or genetic counselor recommends such action and the parents refuse, should the parents be liable for the wrongful life of their child? The availability of the technologies largely defines the options as well as the alternative which is perceived by the community as most responsible.

SUMMARY: HUMAN GENETIC AND REPRODUCTIVE INTERVENTION

The technologies of human genetics and reproduction raise critical policy dilemmas that increasingly require public attention. On the one hand, these innovations promise to alleviate the individual and social costs of genetic disease and give us more control over the destiny of future generations. They allow us to alter the givens concerning what it means to be a human being. On the other hand, widespread use of these technologies expands considerably the ability to label and categorize individuals according to precise genetic factors. There is the danger of altering our definition of humanity so as to minimize the "human" aspects. This capacity to predetermine the sex of progeny, to select the frozen embryo that best meets one's expectation for a child, and to utilize DNA probes to identify persons with "undesirable" characteristics can easily dehumanize us, despite giving the appearance of expanding individual choice. Clearly, these technologies dramatize the ethical dimensions of any political decisions made in this area.

Increasingly, there are questions as to what role the government should play in setting liability, safety, and confidentiality standards for reproduction enterprises. Should responsibility for monitoring and regulating these practices be delegated to the medical community, specialized professional associations, or individual hospitals and clinics, or is there a need for state intervention to ensure certain minimal standards of safety, efficacy, and privacy? The debate over who regulates the burgeoning reproduction industry is bound to heighten because of the trends discussed here. Moreover, the results of current governmental forays into these innovations, by courts, legislatures, and other bodies, will intensify the controversy over what should be done and by whom.

To date, government reaction to dilemmas of human reproduction has been piecemeal and often contradictory. Because of the inability and/or unwillingness of legislatures to make clear policy initiatives, in large part reproductive policy is being made through common law. One of the fastest growing areas of tort law centers on procreation (see chapter 5), and although the courts largely might be acting responsibly, they do not seem capable of making rational, consistent policy in an area as complex as human reproduction. State statutes, as they exist, result in a haphazard, inconsistent policy framework across the states. National regulatory guidelines of some form are needed to help shape responsibly the growing human fertility intervention services now being undertaken in the United States. Not surprisingly, countries with national health services have been more active toward that end.

CHAPTER THREE

Applying These Techniques: Commercialization of Human Reproduction

*I*N CHAPTER 1, I made the assertion that one of the most troubling trends in human reproductive technology is the growing
commercialization of it. The rapid emergence of the demand for
these innovations has drawn increasing attention from investors,
many of whom are involved in the development of the specific
techniques. Although we as a society place considerable emphasis
on the marketplace as a broker of demands and supply of goods
and services, there are many potential dangers in the privatization
of these technologies. They include: (1) the commodification of
children as products of more and more sophisticated intervention
methods; (2) the intrusion of the profit motive into something as
special and human as procreation; and (3) the potential exploitation of very vulnerable and often desperate consumers.

Barbara Katz Rothman (1986:2) sees reproductive technology

developments as illustrating a broader movement toward commodification of life—toward treating people and parts of people as commodities:

> The new technology of reproduction is building on this commodification. Rather than buying whole bodies, we can now buy the parts. Sperm is relatively cheap. . . . Egg donations are being done only on an experimental basis now: will they eventually become purchasable too? And what of embryo transplants. . . . How long will it be before human embryos, like some animal embryos, are up for sale?

Moreover, Rothman contends that genetic counseling serves the function of quality control in an ever strengthened marketplace of human reproduction.

This chapter focuses attention on several vivid examples of this trend toward commercialization of human reproductive technologies. The development of for-profit sperm banks, the proliferation of private IVF clinics, and the emergence of surrogate mother enterprises, I argue, are but the first wave of a more expansive marketplace in human procreation. In fact, a second, more venturesome wave of marketing has already begun and is reflected in the development and marketing of sex preselection kits and genetic screening devices. This chapter analyzes the policy problems inherent in this movement of fertility services into a market framework including: deception in marketing (i.e., exaggerated efficacy and safety); inaccessibility to persons without ability to pay; obscuring of lines between therapeutic and experimental applications; and exploitation of various parties involved. In each case, there appears to be a growing need for public intervention of some form to protect potential consumers of these services as well as the public purse.

ARTIFICIAL INSEMINATION: THE EMERGENCE OF COMMERCIAL INVOLVEMENT IN HUMAN REPRODUCTION

As noted in chapter 2, the most widely used form of technology-mediated reproduction today is artificial insemination, the introduction of semen from either the husband or an unrelated donor by mechanical means into a woman's uterus in an effort to achieve conception. Because of its widespread use and because of related developments in cryopreservation, commercialization of AID represents the first wave of human reproduction for profit. The scarcity of adoptable infants, in combination with recent innovations in sperm banking and the increasing occurrence of infertility, promises to expand the market for AID services.

Sperm Donors: On Consignment

It has been suggested by Annas (1980) that the term "donor" as applied to AID is a misnomer. Virtually all the practitioners responding to the Curie-Cohen (1979) survey paid for semen samples: 90 percent paid between $20 and $35 per ejaculate with 7 percent paying more, up to a high of $100. Annas (1980:6) opts for the term "sperm vendor" and argues that the consent form which is signed is, in actuality, a contract in which the sperm vendor agrees to deliver a product for pay. Although there is merit in the label "vendor," the term "consignor" is used here to refer to those men who "transfer their semen to another's charge or custody." This transfer normally will involve a fee, though it need not.

Also, the transfer might be made to a sperm bank for later transfer to one or more recipient women. In this latter instance, the consignor will likely get paid, although motivation other than money might become more common in those few sperm banks which exist primarily for eugenic purposes. The Repository for Germinal Choice, for instance, depends upon Nobel laureates and other men who contribute their sperm for eugenic or egocentric reasons, not monetary gain. The reemergence of a eugenic interest in AID, coupled with the increased competitiveness of sperm banks, could lead to an escalation of the costs of semen samples. For instance, what price would the sperm of an athlete superstar bring, or a great pianist, or a rock star? Given the myriad of ways in which celebrities are sold through the American media marketplace, what could represent more personal commitment to one's hero than to carry his baby? Perhaps the ultimate in "selling" the star is possible today, and the laws in many states would absolve the sperm consignor of paternal responsibility.

The potential applications of AID have been extended considerably by the introduction of technologies designed to freeze and preserve sperm at low temperatures for extended time periods. Although the concept of cryobanks for human semen was first

proposed in 1866, it was not until 1953 that a successful and practical cryopreservation technique for human sperm was introduced.
At that time the semen was frozen and stored in dry ice at minus
76°C. Over the next decade, the effects of cryopreservation on subsequent fertilization and pregnancies were evaluated and new
freezing procedures investigated. Over this period less than 25
births were reported from the use of frozen sperm.

Commercial Cryobanking and AID

Since 1964, more advanced and automated methods have been
devised and substantial research has supported the safety and efficacy of cryobanking. The most common method of cryopreservation today is the immersion of semen in liquid nitrogen:

> Cans with ampules containing semen are suspended over the vapors
> of liquid nitrogen, the freezing temperature of which is -80°C. The
> cans are then submerged in the liquid nitrogen container, lowering
> the temperature to -196.5°C (Barkay and Zuckerman 1980:184).

Although the initial development of cryobanking was inhibited by
warnings from the American Public Health Association and Planned
Parenthood-World Population in the early 1970s, research confirm-
ing its safety defused some opposition and increased appreciation
of the potential beneficial uses. At present, semen bank facilities
are available in many cities (see table 3.1). According to the American Association of Tissue Banks, there are over seventy commercial, nonprofit, and university-based sperm banks in the United
States. The establishment of the first semen banks was based primarily on the expectation that millions of men would elect to store
their semen prior to undergoing vasectomy for fertility insurance,
an expectation largely unrealized to date (Sherman 1980:97). Interestingly, after an initial surge in the establishment of commercial
banks in the early 1970s, there was a substantial downturn shortly
after, largely the result of inaccurate market predictions and scientific constraints (Frankel 1979:93). Since 1979, however, there has
been a gradual but continuous growth in the number of semen
cryobanking facilities.

Other uses of cryobanking include timed multiple inseminations
for AIH and AID; storage pooling and concentration of sperm for
AIH; retention of fertilizing capacity in absence, death, or hazard

TABLE 3.1. Selected Human Semen Cryobanks in the United States

Name	Location
Astarte Lab, Inc.	Jacksonville, Ala.
University of Arkansas Semen Cryobank	Little Rock
Arizona Fertility Institute	Phoenix
Southwest Fertility Center	Phoenix
Northern California Cryobank	Charmichael, Cal.
Repository for Germinal Choice	Escondido, Cal.
California Cryobank, Inc.	Los Angeles
Tyler Medical Clinic	Los Angeles
The Life Bank	Manhattan Beach, Cal.
Sperm Bank of Northern California	Oakland
Fertility Institute of Southern California	Santa Ana, Cal.
Zygon Laboratory	Tarzana, Cal.
Western Cryobank	Colorado Springs
Washington Fertility Study Center	Washington, D. C.
Paces Cryobank and Fertility Service	Atlanta
Xytex Corporation	Augusta
Cryo Laboratory Facility	Chicago
Rush Medical College	Chicago
Reproductive Resources	Kenner, La.
International Cryogenics, Inc.	Birmingham, Mich.
Ann Arbor Reproductive Medicine	Ypsilanti
Cryogenic Laboratory, Inc.	Roseville, Minn.
University of Missouri	Columbia Mo.
Midwest Fertility Foundation and Laboratory	Kansas City, Mo.
Genetic Sperm Bank	Omaha
Biogenics Corporation	Irvington, N. J.
Idant Laboratory	New York
Andrology Laboratory	Rochester
Hoxworth Blood Center	Cincinnati
Andrology Laboratory	Cleveland
Cleveland Clinic Sperm Bank	Cleveland
Jefferson Semen Bank	Philadelphia
Pennsylvania Cryobank, Inc.	Philadelphia
Drs. Sparr, Stephens, and Associates	Dallas
Fairfax Cyrobank	Fairfax, Va.
Reproductive Genetics Group	Seattle
University of Wisconsin	Madison
Rocky Mountain Cryobank	Jackson, Wy.

exposure of husband; or on-demand AID with a wide selection of genetic traits. Cryobanking can also be used to freeze the semen of patients with specific forms of cancer such as Hodgkin's disease before they undergo necessary cytotoxic chemotherapy or radiation therapy. It has been found that radiation therapy to the abdominal area scatters to the testes and induces azoospermia, the absence of live sperm (Chapman 1979). According to Begent (1982:161): "The prolonged survival of substantial proportion of young men with certain malignancies appears to justify semen storage before treatment when it is known that therapy is likely to render them azoospermatic." Cryobanking has advantages over fresh sperm in that it is always available independent of the donor's availability and it offers recipients a relatively wide choice of donor characteristics.

A final motivation for the use of cryopreservation is to establish eugenic programs that store semen of donors selected for their particular characteristics. The first and most publicized of eugenically motivated sperm banks is the nonprofit Repository for Germinal Choice (RGC). The founder, Robert K. Graham, is a California tycoon and friend of the late Hermann J. Muller, a Nobel laureate in genetics in 1946, who advocated sperm banks for famous, exceptional men. The RGC has semen samples of five Nobel prize winners and other men of note. The clientele of this cryobank are women selected for their high intelligence who desire to have children by men with similarly high intelligence. Without doubt, this use of cryobanking is the most controversial. Despite this, as of 1987, 37 children had been born through sperm provided by the RGC.

Despite some continuing concern over the possibility of long-term genetic damage to the sperm during freezing and the decreased fertilization capacity of frozen sperm, its use for AID is widespread. By 1988, the number of births from frozen sperm totaled over 30,000. Most practitioners (74 percent) who use frozen sperm obtain it from commercial sperm banks (OTA 1988b:43). The need for a somewhat greater number of inseminations to achieve pregnancy is outweighed by the convenience of frozen sperm because the donor need not be physically present to provide the sample. Also, the freezing aspect tends to depersonalize the process of AID, making it more acceptable for some people. More importantly, the use of frozen sperm allows for more thorough screening of donors and of the sperm sample directly. This fact has become crucial in light of the transmission of HIV from donors to children born through AID. Because infection from the AIDS virus sometimes takes months to show up as antibodies in the blood, a three-month quarantine of the sperm is considered essential to permit donor testing before the sperm is used. As a result, the American Fertility Society recently called for the use of frozen sperm in all AID procedures.

> Under the present circumstances the use of fresh sperm for donor insemination is no longer warranted . . . all frozen specimens should be quarantined for 180 days and the donor retested and found to be seronegative for HIV before the specimen is released. (American Fertility Society 1988:211)

THE MARKETING OF HUMAN EMBRYOS

By far the most publicized method of mediated reproduction is in vitro fertilization (IVF). Although AID continues to enjoy considerably wider application, IVF has sparked considerably more debate (Bonnicksen 1989). Books and articles about IVF written for mass consumption are now commonplace. Although it is no longer front page news, the production of "test-tube" babies continues to be of salient interest to the American public. It is hard to believe that as late as 1978 references to IVF were most common, not in the press, but in science fiction literature. The birth of Louise Brown in England, July 1978, triggered an avalanche of research activity and public interest in reproduction technology that has yet to ebb. The rapid proliferation of mediated reproduction services and techniques can be traced to that single success, which came after seven years of uncelebrated attempts to attain that goal.

The demand for IVF services is sizable and growing. Gold (1985:28) reports that the Norfolk clinic alone has a waiting list of more than 8000 names, a sixteen-year backlog. Not surprisingly, commercialization has emerged in this highly lucrative market. Bonnicksen (1985:22) suggests that this rapid growth of IVF services "increases the possibility that clinics will be improperly staffed or will not maintain rigorous quality control." Commercialization opens the door to potential exploitation and to the acceptance of patients that should not be treated by this method but who are desperate and have the up front money necessary to initiate the process.

According to Raymond (1988:464), the commercialization process with IVF has already begun in earnest, "Buffeted by the pressures of commercial interests and near-desperate patients searching for a technological miracle, the technique has become a major player in an increasingly lucrative fertility market." There is no doubt that reproductive technology has tremendous potential to be profit making. The estimated potential clientele, according to Bonnicksen (1989:25) is one million persons with an estimated income in 1990 of $2 billion. In 1987, $70 million went into attempts at IVF, which translates into 7000 couples paying an average of $10,000 each for IVF. Of the 190 IVF centers, about one-fourth currently are private for-profit clinics (Raymond 1988:464). Increasingly, these private centers use aggressive marketing techniques in order to create for themselves reputations as centers of excellence. At least two chains of IVF centers have been established and private clinics "recruit patients by mass mailings to gynecologists, advertisements in professional journals, and packaged brochures" (Bonnicksen 1989:26).

Controversy over the incursion of commercial enterprises in IVF surfaced at an annual meeting of the American Fertility Society. Questions over whether and how the performance of IVF centers should be monitored elicited sharp disagreement even within the IVF community. Geoffrey Sher, co-director of the Northern Nevada Fertility Center in Reno, which showed a profit in performing about 200 procedures in 1987, argues there is "no sin in being profitable" provided you deliver what you promise. In contrast, Richard Marrs, director of the IVF clinic at Good Samaritan Medical Center, contends that an emphasis on making a profit hinders basic research, because for-profit firms pay little attention to the mundane but essential research. Howard Jones, founder of the Norfolk clinic, adds that those who are making a profit on IVF are "cutting corners somewhere" (Raymond 1988:464). It is likely that reduction in essential counseling and screening services will follow such efforts to cut costs.

Other IVF experts are skeptical of the tendency of some business interests to make IVF the treatment of choice and raise questions as to how success rates are presented to the consumer public. Not surprisingly, many centers use those measures which are most favorable to their interest but which are misleading. For instance, many IVF clinics have yet to register a live birth but, using optimistic figures, are offering IVF to couples. Although clients of the most

experienced clinics can expect a 12 to 20 percent birth rate per
cycle, the national success rate is only about 5 percent. Furthermore, in the United States, over 50 percent of IVF births have
occurred in three clinics (the Jones Clinic in Norfolk, the Cedar-
Sinai Center while Richard Marrs was there as director, and the
Pacific Fertility Center in San Francisco).

The wide variation in success rates, as measured by the percentage of procedures that result in live births, is illustrated clearly by
the findings of a survey conducted by the House Subcommittee on
Regulation, Business Opportunities, and Energy in 1989 (table 3.2).
Of the 145 clinics using IVF and/or GIFT in 1987, only a small
percentage (14 for IVF and 22 for GIFT) reported birth rates of over
15 percent. Significantly, 23 percent of those using IVF and 34
percent of those using GIFT had not yet achieved a birth. The use
of conflicting criteria for defining success rates by IVF clinics, along
with the variance in selection criteria, raise critical policy questions concerning consumer education and public access to this
critical data. Although the optimal means of monitoring individual
clinic operations would be a voluntary accrediting system, attempts by the American Fertility Society have met with resistance.
The national registry of IVF centers continues to depend on voluntary compliance. Moreover, over one-third of the IVF centers are
not participants in the registry.

From interviews with IVF specialists, Raymond (1988:465) found
agreement that physicians advise couples seeking fertility treatment to ask the following questions:

TABLE 3.2. Success Rates for IVF and GIFT

Reported Birth Rate	Percentage of Clinics Performing	
	IVF	GIFT
over 20%	4	16
16–20%	10	6
11–15%	15	8
5–10%	24	3
less than 5%	8	3
0	23	34
no treatments	16	30

1. What is that center's pregnancy rate and how is pregnancy defined? The rate should include only pregnancies verified by ultrasound, not so-called chemical pregnancies.
2. What is the pregnancy rate for other women with similar diagnosis?
3. How many babies are produced per procedure? Per egg retrieval?
4. Does the clinic offer other fertility therapies?
5. How many cycles are attempted per patient, with what likelihood of success over that period?
6. Is the program community-based or a referral center?

Because couples anticipating IVF or other treatments for infertility are at the mercy of the medical community for information, they must have access to objective, consistent data of this nature. If the quickly emerging IVF industry fails to guarantee access to such information, government regulation might be necessary for consumer protection. In a recent survey (Bonnicksen and Blank 1988), IVF directors were found to favor government involvement which supports their interests (i. e., state legislation mandating insurance coverage for IVF) but reject those forms of government involvement which are perceived as interference with their practice (i. e., state mandated reporting or licensing regulations).

This already substantial demand for IVF services is certain to intensify as IVF pregnancy success rates increase and its availability to the population expands. As is illustrated by the passage of the 1987 Massachusetts law mandating insurance coverage for IVF and other fertility services, pressures are mounting for insurance companies to cover all or part of the costs of the procedure. Although the Massachusetts law specifically exempts payment by Medicaid for individuals without insurance, claims for such coverage are inevitable. Moreover, as the costs are reimbursed in whole or in part by third-party payers, the demand for such services will intensify.

Although selection criteria vary among clinics, normally they include the following elements:

1. Couples must be legally married and in excellent health.
2. Infertility cannot be corrected by surgery or other treatment.
3. The woman must be under 35 years of age (although an increasing number accept women up to or over 40 years of age).
4. The menstrual cycle must be regular, the uterus and ovaries normal and accessible to laparoscopy.

As IVF becomes a routinized procedure, pressures are being exerted to offer it to single women. A recent note in the *Harvard Law Review* (1985) concludes that the rights of reproductive autonomy guaranteed by the Supreme Court extends to the use of IVF and that the legal right of the woman to seek treatment for infertility outweighs any state interest to protect her health or the health of the embryo.

A most controversial scenario involving IVF occurs when a couple undergoes IVF and has the embryo implanted in another woman's uterus to be carried to term, thus complicating the current notion of surrogate motherhood. This procedure would most likely include payment to the carrying mother for womb space for nine months. Although this raises substantial legal and ethical questions, it is analogous to surrogate motherhood by artificial insemination, which is the method now used in surrogate motherhood applications such as Baby M. Although there are rare medical indications for IVF in a surrogate, such as a case where a woman has functioning ovaries but a diseased or absent uterus and cannot carry a fetus, this more likely represents a nonclinical use of IVF for reasons of convenience, career, or other personal reasons.

Frozen Embryo Transfer

In the summer of 1984, worldwide attention focused on the fate of two frozen embryos in Australia that became "orphaned" when their "mother" and her husband were killed in an airplane crash. Debate abounded over the legal status of the embryos (could they claim part of the estate?), the proper disposition of them, and the appropriate person to decide their ultimate fate. This situation also raised a furor among groups opposed to the procedure itself. This case escalated to a political issue when right-to-life groups lobbied the Victoria parliament to void an ethics commission decision to allow the embryos to be destroyed. Ultimately, and quietly, the embryos were transferred to the wombs of "adoptive" mothers, where they failed to result in pregnancies.

The initial research program in the use of frozen embryos was located at Monash University in Melbourne in the early 1980s. In 1986, IVF Australia, Ltd., a corporation based at Monash University, opened its first clinic in New York City and thus exported this technique to the U.S., where a moratorium on public funding of frozen embryo research had impeded its development. As of 1987, several hundred pregnancies had been achieved using eggs that were fertilized in vitro and then frozen and stored before being transferred to the woman's uterus. In March 1988, IVF Australia held a party in New York City at which 54 of the 169 babies conceived at that clinic, including five pairs of twins, turned out to celebrate.

The process of cryopreservation of embryos is similar to that employed in sperm banking. Although there continues to be a variation in specific technique, commonly embryos are frozen upon reaching the two- to eight-cell stage of division (Friedler, Giudice, and Lamb, 1988). They are gradually cooled to minus 196°C and stored in liquid nitrogen until the strategic time in the recipient woman's cycle, when they are thawed and placed in the uterus. A recent study (Cohen et al. 1988) found that, depending on the cell stage, up to 81 percent of embryos survive cryostorage.

The use of frozen embryos has the advantage that multiple eggs can be retrieved from the woman's ovaries at one time. One or several embryos can be transferred to the uterus while the others are frozen for future use should the pregnancy not take. This procedure obviates the need to go through the difficult egg-retrieval process each time and reduces the cost to about one tenth of what the original procedure costs. In other words, for those many women who must go through a series of IVF attempts, the cost of all tries after the first, which includes egg retrieval, is reduced to approximately $500 each.

The frozen embryo technique is also useful for those women who, because of ovary dysfunction, are unable to produce their own eggs and desire to be the recipient of another woman's embryo. Although IVF without cryopreservation could be used to achieve this end, synchronization of the cycles of the donor and recipient women is very difficult. A frozen embryo, however, could be thawed and transferred to the recipient at the most appropriate time, thus increasing considerably the rate of pregnancy achieved. Despite the opposition to the notion of frozen embryos by many segments of U.S. society, these advantages of cost effectiveness and flexibility undoubtedly will motivate the use of this procedure in IVF programs, and will expand substantially the options of infertile couples. Importantly, this capacity will also encourage the establishment of commercial embryo banks analogous to existing sperm banks. In a recent survey of U.S. IVF directors (Bonnicksen and Blank 1988), all respondents indicated that they planned to use frozen embryos in their practice within five years. Currently, about half of the women undergoing IVF have embryos frozen. This rapid expansion in the use of cryopreservation of embryos is reflected by data indicating that American clinics froze 289 embryos in 1985, 824 in 1986, and 3715 in 1987 (Lieber 1989:77).

EMBRYOS FOR RESEARCH:
A CONTINUING CONTROVERSY

One of the questions often raised concerning the use of IVF or embryo lavage is what becomes of the embryos that are not implanted in the recipient woman's uterus. Especially when used in conjunction with superovulation, these techniques produce many "spare" embryos that can either be destroyed or saved. Controversy is heated over either of these options, but more often it is directed at the fate of those embryos which are not destroyed. They could be frozen for future insemination attempts or, alternately, they could be used for research purposes.

There is a variety of laboratory uses to which IVF might be put. Instead of implanting the embryo in the uterus, one could employ IVF without subsequent embryo transfer, thereby creating the embryos specifically for research purposes. Nonclinical applications of IVF include the production of embryos to: (1) develop and test contraceptives; (2) investigate abnormal cell growth; (3) determine certain causes of cancer; and (4) study the development of chromosomal abnormalities. Other potential genetic uses of the embryos include: (1) attempts at altering gene structures; (2) preimplantation repair of genetic defects; and (3) preimplantational screening for chromosomal abnormalities and genetic defects. Finally, research on artificial placentas depends on the availability of such human materials.

The goals of embryo research are broad in scope and the promised gains in knowledge concerning infertility, contraception, malignant tumors, teratogens, chromosomal abnormalities, abnormal cell growth, and cell differentiation are impressive. Short (1978) suggests that another area of embryo research should be the assessment of IVF itself to determine whether that process produces a higher incidence of embryonic abnormalities than the conventional method of reproduction. If IVF or cryopreservation of embryos does in fact lead to an excess of abnormalities (of which there is presently no evidence), it would be preferable to discover that excess in the laboratory rather than at the time of amniocentesis or birth. Conversely, Biggers (1978) argues that a suitable animal model can be found for most questions concerning human reproduction and should be used where at all possible; valuable human ova and embryos should not be used for laboratory research unless there is no reasonable alternative to human research.

In February 1982, Steptoe and Edwards, who four years earlier reported the first live birth through IVF, created another tumult by announcing plans to freeze "spare" human eggs or embryos for clinical or laboratory use. After selection of the most normal-looking eggs for IVF and embryo transfer, the extra eggs could either be retained for a second try at pregnancy later or destroyed. Grobstein notes that animal studies demonstrate that freezing stops egg development with minimal damage and that, when thawed, a very high proportion undergo normal development. In addition, Edwards asserted (Williams and Stevens 1982:314) that these spare embryos "can be very useful. They can teach us things about early human life which will help that patient and other patients."

At the base of the debate over the acceptability of embryo research is the moral status of the early human embryo. Is such research compatible with the respect due the embryo and, if so, do the potential benefits of such research outweigh the potential adverse consequences? If these questions are answered affirmatively, then attention shifts to proper standards which should be instituted to secure prior consent of the ovum donors, set criteria for establishing the need for human research, and ensure a consideration of weighing risks against benefits in specific research proposals.

Kass (1978) contends that one must distinguish between embryos deliberately created for research purposes and untransferred embryos remaining after fertilization of multiple ova and insertion of only one to the uterus. He concludes that embryos should not be created solely for laboratory research purposes, nor should invasive or manipulative research be performed on already existing human embryos. (The danger in proscribing creation of embryos specifically for research purposes, I feel, is that it will escalate the use of superovulation prior to IVF or embryo lavage so that enough "spares" are available for research. Under these conditions, I envision a market in scarce embryos.) Because of the continuity in embryonic and fetal development and the potential viability of the early human embryo if it is transferred at the proper time, Kass (1978:11) contends that any other policy would symbolize the belief that early human embryos are nothing but "things or mere stuff." Kass clearly advocates a position which would prohibit human embryo research. Instead of transferring spare embryos to women other than the donor or using them for laboratory research, Kass expresses a clear preference for allowing untransferred embryos to die.

Grobstein (1982) concludes that "human cells, tissues, and organs that have no reasonable prospect of possessing or developing sentient awareness" are "human materials rather than human beings or persons." He contends (1982:6) that scientific evidence suggests that up to the eight-cell stage, at least, a multicellular individual is not present. The cells continue to act as individual cells rather than cell-parts of multicellular individual. Because individuals are usually defined as multicellular it is "difficult to maintain scientifically that a person has come into existence prior to the eight-cell stage." Grobstein argues that because the entire preimplantation period is a preindividual stage in a developmental sense, at least to that point, safety of the procedure ought to be the prime concern and errors with human materials are not to be tolerated easily.

For Gorovitz (1978) the primary criterion for determining the moral status of the human embryo is sentience, which occurs after about eight to ten weeks of gestation. He contends that the status of the embryo "is not equivalent to that of a person, a child, an infant, or a fetus," at least from the point of development where a capacity for even "primitive sentience" is present. That is the stage where the conceptual line between a morally "nonprotected" and "protected" status would occur. This line for Gorovitz (1978:28) is "rather close to the point where cell differentiation begins, rather far from the capacity for independent survival." According to the Ethics Advisory Board report (1979:15):

> If one extrapolates from Gorovitz's views on embryonic status, one concludes that he would approve of any type of research procedure on the human embryo, provided only that the research terminated prior to the onset of embryonic or fetal sentience and that other canons of research ethics. . .were carefully followed.

Although there has been considerable discussion on the moral aspects of embryo research, focusing primarily on differing conceptions of the moral status of the developing organism, the legal status of the preimplanted embryo also has been raised. In *Del Zio v. Presbyterian Hospital* (1978), a jury awarded $50,000 for emotional distress following the intentional destruction of a culture containing gametes of the plaintiffs. This suggests that although the early embryo is not a legal person (*Roe v. Wade*, 1973), the special interests of the donors embodied in the embryo gives it a legal value, if not a legal status of some sort. Despite this single decision, Flannary et al. (1978:88) conclude it is unlikely that the courts will ultimately extend the concept of "wrongful death" to include intentional destruction of a preimplanted embryo. Similarly, Katz (1978:21–25) concludes that it is unlikely that the destruction of preimplantation embryos will fall within homicide or anti-abortion statutes. Reilly (1977:214), however, contends that this legal status of the embryo must be defined so that laboratory technicians and clinicians will be aware of their legal responsibilities regarding the material and products of their work. At present, approximately 24 states have fetal research laws (see discussion in chapter 5), many of which could be used to proscribe research on human embryos, but which have not yet been tested in the courts. Other legal issues (Seibel 1988:834) surrounding frozen embryos concern the authority to dispose of the embryo, the length of storage, posthumous use, inheritance rights, and family relations, including custody of the embryos after divorce such as in the Tennessee case noted earlier. Whether used for clinical or research purposes, cryopreservation of human embryos will engender intense debate.

Summary: Marketing Human Embryos

Human embryos are fast becoming a commodity, whether for use to circumvent infertility or for a multitude of research purposes. Increasingly, technological innovations allow us to intervene in the procreative process at the preconception and conception stages. More importantly, current trends demonstrate a growing demand for technology-mediated conception that introduces third parties into what, until recently, was a private matter between a man and a woman. These third parties include an ever-expanding array of specialists and professionals who provide essential services as well as the consigners of germ material. They include researchers who are primarily interested in obtaining human germ material and embryos for experimental rather than clinical purposes. Significantly, they also include entrepreneurs who anticipate, correctly I believe, a potentially lucrative market for their services and products.

At the very least, these patterns necessitate a close monitoring of the possible social consequences of the commodification of human embryos. We must reevaluate what social priorities ought to take precedence. Do we want to facilitate the marketing of human embryos and, if so, for what purposes: research, clinical, or eugenic? What constraints, if any, should be imposed on such endeavors and what protections should be given the various parties to them? It seems that the government must have some role in this area, but what should it entail? Is the current pattern of individual state prohibition in response to specific interest groups the answer or is national government action warranted? Without doubt, these questions are certain to create intense debate and they should. Unfortunately, the proliferation of new techniques and their widening usage is outpacing our efforts to deal with their policy ramifications.

IVF AND SELECTIVE REDUCTION OF FETUSES

One complication in the current use of IVF and fertility drugs is the increased number of pregnancies complicated by multiple gestation. As noted earlier, the practice of transferring multiple embryos in order to maximize the chances of pregnancy through IVF leads to a heightened rate of multiple pregnancies when many of the embryos implant. In such pregnancies, the adverse outcome is directly proportional to the number of fetuses, largely because of severely premature delivery. Hobbins (1988:1062) describes a recent case of delivery of quintuplets at Yale-New Haven Hospital:

> One baby died of respiratory distress syndrome within two days. One baby required operations for necrotizing enterocolitis and is also blind. One baby required a shunt for posthemorrphagic hydrocephalus; another had chronic lung disease. The fifth baby had neonatal seizures due to perinatal eschemia. The total cost of neonatal care was $300,000. This did not include the many days of antepartum hospitalization required to keep the mother out of labor.

According to Hobbins (1988:1062), multiple gestation represents the "down side" of induced ovulation and IVF.

Ironically, one option now being used to deal with multifetal pregnancies directly caused by reproductive mediation technologies is the selective reduction of fetuses to increase the chances of delivery of infants mature enough to survive without suffering irreversible damage caused by marked prematurity. Berkowitz et al. (1988) recently reported their experience in selective reduction of twelve multifetal pregnancies. Two patients had each conceived six fetuses, one had five, five had four, and four had triplets. By using one of two methods (transvaginal aspiration of the amniotic fluid from the lowest sacs or transabdominal injection of potassium chloride into the fetal hearts) between nine and thirteen weeks gestation, Berkowitz and associates reduced the number of fetuses to two in eleven cases and to three in one pregnancy. Seven of the patients delivered healthy twins, one had a healthy single infant, and four had no liveborn births. According to Hobbins (1988:1063):

> The total number of infants born alive in the 12 study pregnancies (15 of 49) may not be very different from what would be expected in a similar group of patients who did not have the operation. However, 13 of the 15 survivors were delivered at 34 weeks or more of gestation, when morbidity is appreciably lower.

Berkowitz et al. (1988:1046) do raise the difficult issues associated with their procedure, pointing out that it is all the more difficult because patients who conceive multiple fetuses as a result of infertility treatment are desperate to have children. The decision to undergo this procedure, which might result in the loss of the entire pregnancy, is a painful one for these patients. Extensive counseling concerning the risks is crucial, as is the need for better data on the risk/benefit relation according to the number of fetuses. It seems clear that women carrying four or more fetuses are at substantial risk for adverse outcomes and are likely candidates for selective reduction. Triplet gestations are more problematic. Interestingly, however, Berkowitz et al. (1988:1046) report that in each of the four pregnancies in which they reduced triplets to twins, the patients had decided to terminate the entire pregnancy if selective reduction was not available to them.

Under *Roe v. Wade* and abortion on demand in the first trimester, there is no legal problem in selective reduction. A basic ethical issue surrounding this procedure is whether it is justifiable to reduce the number of fetuses in order to lower the unspecified risk to all fetuses. Even with sophisticated neonatal intensive care facilities, the chances of salvaging healthy infants in patients with five or more fetuses without use of selective reduction are poor. But for many persons there is still the nagging issue of killing fetuses so that the risk to others is reduced. Also, because the procedure is in effect random, the healthier fetuses might be aborted. Persons opposed to abortion obviously find this procedure morally repugnant. Those persons who find abortion acceptable under specific circumstances must deal with this difficult concept of sacrificing some fetuses so that others can survive. Despite his concern with the ethical problems, in his editorial comment on the Berkowitz study, Hobbins (1988:1063) concludes that this "remarkable study will be encouraging to couples faced with an overabundance of conceptuses."

The use of frozen embryos and other advances in IVF might well reduce the number of multiple gestations by removing the need to transfer large numbers of embryos. On the other hand, the proliferation of commercial fertility clinics offering IVF and the resulting pressures to maximize success rates could lead to an increase in multiple gestation. In any case, this dimension further complicates the social impact of IVF and other fertility mediating technologies. It also raises substantial questions concerning the psychological ramifications for women undergoing these procedures in the hopes of having a healthy child, because it introduces yet another difficult decision she might be forced to face.

SURROGATE MOTHERHOOD: WOMBS FOR RENT

Artificial insemination, in combination with cryopreservation techniques for freezing germ material, in vitro fertilization, and an array of innovations in embryo transfer mean that, with increased frequency, the woman carrying the fetus is not necessarily the genetic or biological mother. More critical, however, is the variety of unique applications of these technologies such as surrogate motherhood (SM) where a couple (or individual) contracts with a woman to carry a child to term for them. Surrogate mother contracts have multiplied since 1980 because many couples with infertility problems see SM as the answer. Although the first reported surrogate birth is in the biblical account of Abraham siring a son with his wife's maid Hagar when Sarah was unable to bear children, the first publicized surrogate birth via artificial insemination occurred in Kentucky in 1980. Since that time, it is estimated that 750–1000 births have resulted from the use of surrogate mothers in the United States (New York State Task Force 1988:25).

Under the most straightforward SM procedure, an infertile woman and her husband enter into an agreement with the surrogate under which she will be artificially inseminated with the sperm of the husband. After fertilization, the surrogate carries the fetus to term. When the baby is born, she relinquishes her rights to it and surrenders it to the couple (or more precisely in some contracts, to the husband of the couple, the genetic father). Usually, but not always, this agreement is a detailed contract which stipulates that the surrogate will receive compensation for her service. The result of this legal procedure is a child for a couple that otherwise would have to undergo more lengthy and possibly unsuccessful adoption proceedings. Surrogate motherhood through AID, also has an added attractiveness to some couples because the child is biologically related to the husband. Although SM entails the use of a clinical procedure, it must be emphasized that it is primarily a legal procedure carried out under the auspices of lawyers.

Reported costs of up to $50,000 for adoption of a healthy newborn certainly contributes to the attractiveness of surrogate programs for some U.S. couples. In most cases, the total cost of a surrogate contract is between $25,000 and $40,000. Of this, it is common for the surrogate mother to receive $10,000 for her services, although figures as high as $50,000 have been offered (figure 3.1). As Field notes: "today it should be possible for some women, if they are sufficiently healthy and attractive, to obtain $75,000 or $100,000, and the current demand for surrogacy may be only incipient" (1988:26). The remainder (between $15,000 and $30,000) goes to the lawyer or firm that arranges the contract. Expenses include counseling of the couple, screening and selection of the surrogate mother, medical expenses through pregnancy and delivery (including prenatal diagnosis), liability insurance, and attorney fees.

As surrogate contracts become commonplace, competition among providers could conceivably lower the cost. It is more likely, however, that as demand escalates the cost of surrogacy will escalate. Unless some consumer protection is provided, exploitation of this demand from less trustworthy surrogate businesses will be manifest in high charges for inadequate service. Most likely, these firms will maximize their profit by reducing needed psychological counseling and screening of all parties to the contract and cutting other less tangible costs, to the detriment of both the couple and the surrogate mother. The question of exploitation of the surrogate by bargaining for lower fees must also be examined carefully by lawmakers in states where surrogate contracts involving payment are allowed. Whatever policy eventually emerges, it is clear that motherhood under these circumstances becomes a business proposition. Procreation here is a commercial endeavor where the various parties (couple, surrogate mother, attorneys, and so forth) are related through legal contracts. Barbara Katz Rothman (1987:4) warns that this practice will encourage "production standards" in pregnancy and result in viewing it as a service, rather than as a relationship between mother and fetus.

At a time when the courts, legislators, and legal profession are beginning to grapple with surrogate motherhood in conjunction with artificial insemination technology, new reproductive options are emerging which complicate the problem considerably. These innovations include IVF, embryo transfer, and embryo adoption.

FIGURE 3.1. Advertisement for Surrogate Mother

Surrogate Mother

We are seeking a surrogate mother to bear a child through artificial insemination. Applicant must be 22-35, tall, trim, intelligent, and stable. Your child will be reared in an outstanding environment.

A successful applicant will be paid $50,000.

Send a resume describing your personal and family background, with a photograph, to

NYR, Box 1663.

As noted above, there is no biological reason why the embryo of a couple, fertilized in vitro, could not be transferred to the uterus of a surrogate mother to carry to term. This could alter the legal status significantly, since all the genetic material comes from the couple. "All" that the surrogate provides here, is the womb for nine months. Similarly, "flushing" out the embryo fertilized in a donor and implanting it in the "adoptive" woman opens new vistas in the field of reproductive law. These new applications, however, do not alter the basic problems caused by placing procreation in a business context.

The legal problems surrounding surrogate motherhood are bound to become more troubling because of the heavy commitment required of the surrogate. Unlike artificial insemination where a donor anonymously sells his semen, SM takes nine months out of a woman's life. In addition to the normal risks of pregnancy which she accepts, her privacy is bound to be invaded by prospective legal parents who might also be the genetic parents. The surrogate mother must be willing to be inseminated by the sperm of a stranger or implanted with the embryo of strangers, carry the fetus to term —often under careful scrutiny of the couple or their legal agent— and turn over the baby to the couple immediately after birth.

The risk to the couple is also high because they must rely totally on the good faith of the surrogate to deliver as promised. According to Harris (1981:952), a couple involved with SM must proceed only with the utmost caution, since no assurance exists that any rights they might have in the child are guaranteed. For Winslade (1981:154), "contracts to bear a child place most of the risks on the prospective adoptive parents" because, in the end, the decision to give up the legal rights to custody of the child rest upon the surrogate mother's informed consent and willingness to honor the agreement after the child is born. A court would be reluctant to hold a surrogate to the specific performance of such a contract, no matter how sound legally, should she refuse to give the child to the biological father and his wife. What if she decides to abort the child against the wishes of the couple or if they attempt to prevent her from smoking or drinking during pregnancy? Also, what should be done if a surrogate such as Mary Beth Whitehead who willingly turns over the child at birth has a change of heart at a later time and demands the return of "her" child? Must the couple go through formal adoption proceedings in order to legitimize the child and protect their custody rights? Or, what if the child is born with a congenital defect and the couple refuses to take custody as stipulated in the agreement? These are but a few of the myriad questions raised by surrogate motherhood that are beginning to be addressed both by case law and statutory law.

Most analysis on this issue so far has centered on whether or not surrogate motherhood contracts are legally permissible and, if so, legally binding. It should be noted that even if such contracts are not declared illegal, they might be judged contrary to public policy and thus be invalid. Moreover, even if they are legally valid, they might not be enforceable, given the variety of questions posited above. As with all applications of reproductive technologies, the legality of surrogate agreements must be interpreted within the constitutional guarantees of the right to bear a child. As noted earlier, childbearing ought to be free from unwarranted or unjustified government intrusion. The basic question is whether or not the government has a compelling interest to intervene. Conversely, does a woman's right to privacy in matters of reproduction include a right to be a surrogate mother, and if so, under what conditions?

Despite the many concerns surrounding surrogate motherhood, payment has emerged as a key issue. In *Doe v. Kelly* (1981), the Michigan Court of Appeals ruled that while a husband and wife could adopt a child via the SM procedure, it would be illegal for them to pay a fee to the surrogate mother. The court held that there was no fundamental right to buy and sell children and that such action violated baby-selling statutes, which in thirty-six states prohibit monetary inducement for adoption (OTA, 1988:281). However, in 1986, the Supreme Court of Kentucky (*Surrogate Parenting Associates, Inc. v. Commonwealth ex rel Armstrong*) held that surrogate parenting contracts do not violate that state's prohibition against purchasing a child for adoption. While the Court concluded that surrogacy was analogous to AI, it emphasized that the contract, though not unlawful, was voidable by the surrogate mother.

In the most authoritative decision to date, the New Jersey Supreme Court (*In re Baby M*, 1988) declared surrogate contracts in that state unenforceable. Although the court granted custody of Baby M. to Dr. Stern, the father, who had contracted with Mary Beth Whitehead to be a surrogate mother of his child, it invalidated surrogate mother contracts. Such contracts violate state adoption laws because of the payment and constitute a form of baby selling. Although the New Jersey decision affects directly only that state, in reaction to the Baby M. case, many state legislatures are moving toward passing statutory prohibitions on surrogate motherhood where money is involved. By March 1988, six states had passed legislation concerning surrogacy (see chapter 5). Moreover, in Congress at least four bills have been introduced that would prohibit commercial surrogacy arrangements. A less-known fact about the Baby M case is that Mary Beth Whitehead and her former husband, Richard Whitehead, reached an out-of-court settlement with the Infertility Center of New York which had brokered the contract. They charged the clinic with fraud and negligence in arranging the contract that ended in this prolonged and bitter custody dispute (*American Medical News* 1988:11).

Legal analysts disagree on whether or not criminal statutes affecting prohibitions of payment ought to be changed. Van Hoften (1981:385), for instance, concludes that the penal code provisions prohibiting payment for the transfer of custody and adoption should not be modified, at least at this stage. Winslade (1981:154) disagrees. He contends that baby-selling statutes were intended to protect poor women from selling their children, as well as to prevent economic exploitation of such babies and adoptive parents. Surrogate motherhood, however, is at variance with the intention of these laws because the woman is not selling a baby already conceived or born, but rather entering into an agreement to have a baby with the purpose of giving it up for adoption.

Winslade (1981:154) sees payment of expenses and a nominal ($10,000) fee to a woman for the inconvenience and risks of childbirth at best "a modest" compensation. Field (1988:26) argues that the most oppressive result of all would be to allow surrogacy but prohibit the payment of any fee. Keane (1980:160) contends that if an individual has a basic constitutional right to procreate by means of a surrogate, there is a question whether any state interest in preventing the buying and selling of surrogate services overrides that fundamental right. Additionally, the surrogate mother would seem to have similar constitutional protection to bear, but not raise, the child. Evidence suggests that while economic motives alone are seldom enough for a woman to enter an SM agreement, 80 percent of actual applicants to be a surrogate mother would require a fee if they were to go through with the procedure (*New York Times* 1981). Given the confusion about payment of fees, Harris (1981:952) concludes that "to avoid jeopardizing the rights of the sponsoring couple, no compensation should be offered or paid to the surrogate."

Still, in most cases on record some fee has been paid to the surrogate mother. The usual method of payment is for the couple to cover prenatal expenses as they come due and place the major portion of the fee in escrow until delivery of the baby. There is at least one report of blackmail attempt by a surrogate mother who threatened to have an abortion unless the couple paid her $7500 (Keane and Breo 1981). Although this seems to be a relatively isolated incident, it reinforces the tentative nature of surrogate agreements. Contrarily, there is also a possibility that this procedure could result in the exploitation of poor women and create a class of surrogate mothers. This possibility, however, could be minimized if the payment were kept modest and the supply of available surrogates was large enough to ensure proper screening. These potentialities, however, do demonstrate a troubling economic aspect which is inherent any time a woman carries a child for another.

Proponents of SM contend that the monetary problems can be reduced substantially with an adequate contract. Katie Brophy, a lawyer from Kentucky involved in a surrogate motherhood through Surrogate Family Services, Inc., proposed a basic contract that has been used by all surrogate mothers thus far in that state. The major purposes of this contract are to protect the confidentiality of all parties, protect the parties against the medical and emotional risks involved, and make appropriate use of expert opinion and guidance at every step along the way. Brophy (1982:264) admits that many provisions of the contract are unenforceable and might be considered void because of a statute or a particular court's view of public policy, but this contract serves at least to appraise the parties to it of the various problems that might arise and to provide contingencies in case they do. The contract presented by Brophy is 25 pages long and very detailed. Included are specifications concerning provisions for amniocentesis, behavior of the surrogate mother during pregnancy, and conditions under which abortion is permitted or required. It also spells out the fees and expenses to be paid, those who will have custody of the child, contingency in case of miscarriage, and contingency suits should either the surrogate mother or the couple breach the contract. Even when a contract is used, Harris (1981:952) recommends that at the birth of the child, with the consent of the surrogate, the couple should go through formal adoption proceedings.

As Bird (1982:24) notes, almost everyone who has had some

involvement in surrogate motherhood agrees that some, if not all, of these issues should be addressed by the legislatures. Mady (1981) argues that legislation is needed to resolve ambiguities in the law resulting from the emergence of these innovations in reproduction. He proposes specific legislation that would affirm the legality of the arrangement, clarify the responsibilities of the parties, and protect the best interests of the child. "Under the proposed legislation, legitimacy questions would be resolved by creating a presumption that the child is the legitimate child" of the couple, "thereby making adoption unnecessary" (Mady 1981:352). Keane and Breo (1981) would remove impediments to the use of surrogate motherhood by statutory change.

Interestingly, surrogate motherhood provides an excellent opportunity to see how successful intense pressures for responsible maternal behavior during pregnancy might be. As noted above, SM contracts often specify in great detail what behavior is expected of the woman during pregnancy including nutrition, prenatal medical care, smoking, drinking, and so forth. Presumably, as SM becomes more common, the interests of the couple in having a healthy baby will intrude severely on the personal autonomy of the surrogate mother. Assuming these SM contracts are recognized in at least some states as binding, what would preclude a cause of action against a surrogate mother who breaches the contract by negligently harming the fetus through failure to provide agreed-upon care during this period? Also, it is possible, though less likely, that the child upon birth could initiate tort action for prenatal injury against the surrogate who carried him or her to term. Conceivably, the adoptive (and possibly genetic) parents would be parties to such a suit against the woman.

Ironically, children born via SM might be the first class of persons with a legal claim for adequate maternal behavior during their prenatal life. Unlike conventionally conceived and carried children, the surrogate mother of these children would be legally bound to provide the best of prenatal care and a safe environment for the fetus. If she failed to do so, not only might she not collect the fee, but she might, in fact, face a lawsuit by the other parties to the contract or by the injured child.

The question of whether the surrogate is being compensated for the inconvenience and risks of pregnancy and out-of-pocket expenses or paid for her baby is certain to remain at the core of the legal controversy over SM. It is unlikely that a woman can be

stopped from having a baby for another party if she so desires—
the problem comes when she is compensated for that action. On
the one hand, it is argued that she is the one who takes the risk and
bears the discomfort of pregnancy and therefore she is the one to
make the decision. This argument also assumes that she has a right
to be compensated for her trouble. In effect, she is renting her
womb for nine months and a just compensation is warranted.

Contrarily, the expansion of surrogate motherhood could result
in a situation where some women become surrogate mothers solely
for economic reasons. One study of surrogate mothers, for instance,
found that approximately 85 percent of the women would not have
entered into the arrangement unless they received a fee (Miller
1983:18). When the incentive is monetary, not one of compassion
for the infertile couple, SM raises several potential problems. First,
it might result in the exploitation of women who find the money
attractive and who are willing to submit to severe restrictions on
their privacy for a year or so under a contract and give up the baby
they carried to term in their body. Another study found that all
thirty women who had babies as surrogates experienced some grief,
some so much so that they sought therapeutic counseling (Parker
1983:117). Although there is no evidence to date of the emergence
of a class bias to SM (i.e., middle class couples contracting with
economically vulnerable women), this danger will heighten as SM
becomes more commonplace.

A second problem is that as the demand for SM increases it will
become more commercialized. At present approximately forty SM
programs are operating in the United States. As noted above, in all
or most of these programs, fees are charged for the legal services
and administration—fees that often total over $10,000 and can
reach $32,000. Because there are no legal guidelines nor regula-
tions for SM and no public controls over these programs, there is
no doubt that some lawyers will establish SM programs solely for
the monetary profits they promise. Annas (1981:24) notes that although legislation on SM is probably premature at present, we
need a "set of agreed-on principles" so that SM has a reasonable
chance of doing more good than harm.

Conversely, Furrow (1984:112) contends that SM has been hin-
dered by legal uncertainties and argues that existing laws and
public policy should not be applied to invalidate surrogate motherhood contracts. He sees significant differences between SM and
the blackmarket trade in babies these statutes were designed to

prevent. He dismisses the policy argument that SM may lead to exploitation of financially needy women, but, if such cases arise, they should be addressed by statutes narrowly defined. Mady (1981) advocates legislation that clarifies the legal ambiguities of SM and reaffirms the legality of a properly drawn and executed surrogate mother contract: contracts in the best interests of all parties including the child. According to Cohen (1984:284) the question raised by surrogate motherhood is considerably broader in its implications.

> Ultimately, these new reproductive technologies may require reanalyzing and rewriting large portions of family law. New definitions of parenthood may be in order. . . . However, no matter what results these new laws and science bring, a natural mother's decision to part with her child at birth should be protected from coercion.

She advocates specific legislation or an explicit judicial determination limiting surrogate contracts by treating the surrogate contract as a revokable prebirth agreement and prohibiting any payment other than actual expenses.

COMMERCIALIZATION OF DNA TESTING

The development of for-profit sperm banks, the proliferation of private IVF clinics, and the emergence of surrogate mother enterprises, are but the first wave of a more expansive marketplace in human procreation. In fact, a second, more venturesome wave of marketing has already begun and is reflected in the development and marketing of sex preselection kits and genetic screening devices. According to Lewis (1987:76):

> Commercialization of genetic-marker technology is imminent, vigorously pursued by several biotechnology firms that are eying the large ready-made market for prenatal screening tests. The specter cast by successful malpractice suits brought against obstetricians who failed to use currently available prenatal diagnostic tests ensures a heavy demand for genetic markers.

Major commercial applications of biotechnology center on the development of new diagnostic and therapeutic products. In addition to the production of human insulin, human growth hormone, and new drugs for individuals with heart disease, rDNA techniques are being used to improve a number of diagnostic tests for infectious diseases. One rapidly emerging set of applications which promises a large market for diagnostic products are tests for common conditions which have a genetic component. As noted earlier, until now most tests for genetic-linked diseases have relied, not on identification of the abnormal gene, but rather on detecting abnormalities in the gene product, such as detection of an abnormal protein coded for by the defective gene.

Rapid advances in molecular probes, however, are altering the givens. *Direct* tests for single-gene disorders depend upon isolation and identification of the disease-causing gene. Similarly, *predictive* tests for polygenic or multifactoral disorders are dependent on the identification of genetic markers that are associated with heightened rates of the disorder. As discussed earlier, considerable strides have been achieved in the development of both direct and predictive tests. California Biotechnology, Inc., for instance, is evaluating the predictive value of RFLPs in detecting susceptibilities to atherosclerosis and hypertension (Hewitt and Holtzman 1988:8).

For both direct and predictive applications, widespread testing is feasible only after development of easy and inexpensive tests. With alpha-fetoprotein tests leading the way, test kits for a variety of disorders and susceptibilities will be developed for use in a physician's office or the home. According to Hewitt and Holtzman (1988:5), "as DNA-based kits are simplified, test kits will be commercially developed and marketed." Companies are likely to develop tests for conditions that have a high incidence in the population. Given the rareness of most single-gene disorders when compared with genetic-linked diseases, commercial efforts are likely to emphasize the latter. This conclusion is borne out by one estimate of the U.S. market for DNA tests in table 3.3. Although single-gene disorders are numerous (over 3500 known), because they are relatively rare, the number of tests per year and thus their market value are limited. In contrast, four common diseases with a genetic component (Alzheimer's, cancer, diabetes, and heart disease) are predicted to account for over 90 percent of the market by as soon as 1992 (*Genetic Technology News* 1986:6–7). Also, these predictions do not include potential tests for genetic susceptibilities to alcoholism, obesity, manic-depression, and so forth which, when developed, will enjoy an unlimited market potential. A survey of biotechnology firms, conducted by the Office of Technology Assessment (OTA:1988), found that approximately 20 percent of the 500 plus companies now involved in biotechnology specialize in diagnostic products. In addition, most major pharmaceutical and diagnostic product companies are involved in such research. Forty-nine percent of the respondents to the OTA survey reported the use of rDNA technology to construct molecular probes with an additional 9 percent planning to do so within the next five years. Twenty companies report developing DNA probes to diagnose genetic disease, including single gene, chromosomal, and multifactoral. Moreover, 23 companies report current or anticipated use of research designed to link RFLPs to specific diseases. Finally, four companies report current or future development of human gene therapy.

TABLE 3.3. DNA Probe Tests for Inherited Diseases—
U.S. Market, 1992

Disease	Number of Tests/yr	Value ($ in millions)
Purely genetic diseases		
Adult polycystic kidney	250,000	7.5
Cystic fibrosis	333,000	10.0
Duchenne muscular dystrophy	333,000	10.0
Familial hypercholesterolemia	250,000	7.5
Familial polyposis	165,000	5.0
Huntington's disease	20,000	0.6
Neurofibromatosis	250,000	7.5
Retinoblastoma	250,000	7.5
Sickle cell anemia	250,000	7.5
Other	500,000	15.0
Subtotal	2,500,000	75.0
Common diseases with a genetic component		
Alzheimer's	1,000,000	30.0
Cancer	12,000,000	360.0
Diabetes	5,000,000	150.0
Heart disease	12,000,000	360.0
Subtotal	30,000,000	900.0
TOTAL	32,500,000	950.0– 1,000.0

SOURCE: *Genetic Technology News* 1986:6–7.

CONCLUSIONS: COMMERCIALIZING
HUMAN REPRODUCTION

These selected examples of the movement toward commercialization of human reproduction raise serious questions as to where we, as a society, are going. On a practical level, as we come to view infertile couples and, indeed, all parents as potential consumers of a growing array of genetic and reproductive technologies and services, we must consider the possibility of regulations designed to protect their interests. As noted earlier, this need is more compelling because many of these persons are desparate and willing to try anything that promises results. To defer fully to the marketplace on matters of reproductive technology is to evade social responsibility.

The transformation of procreation from a matter of intimacy between two persons to yet another market enterprise also raises serious conceptual concerns. When the most private of human endeavors becomes a matter of entrepreneurship, it is imperative that we carefully analyze how this revolution in thinking, as well as technique, affects human relationships. How will this trend alter our views of parental responsibility, of children, and of women? How far can we proceed in this direction without entering a brave new world of procreation as a manufacturing process? While I doubt that our value system will permit wholesale moves toward that end, we must be alert to the potential dangers of these current trends. Chapter 4 examines in more detail the broader social implications of the heightened capacities to design our children.

CHAPTER FOUR

Designing Our Children: At What Cost?

*I*N CHAPTER 1, I argued that the second reproductive revolution, like the first, is having substantial impact on all social structures, especially the family. Together, the technologies introduced here challenge traditional notions of parenthood, the meaning of children, and the relationship between parents and children. Even the concepts of motherhood and fatherhood are undergoing rapid transformation. The expanding array of reproductive interventions forces division of the procreation process into discrete parts, thereby creating or reshaping roles for the many participants. Moreover, the active involvement of many third parties in each stage of procreation removes it from the intimacy of the personal realm to the glare of the public spotlight.

This chapter focuses attention on how reproductive technologies affect the way we view others in society. It analyzes their impact on parenting, family formation, and family dynamics. Although the primary impetus behind the rapid diffusion of these technologies comes from the demands of individual women, some observers place blame on traditional cultural values that overstate the role of motherhood and lead women to equate infertility with a useless life. These technologies have tremendous implications for the way in which women are perceived in society.

Although most attention to date has been directed toward the rights of adults regarding reproduction, it is the children (the products of the technologies) who are most directly affected, because the very availability of the techniques allows for the designing of children to particular specifications. This potentiality, among all others, has the greatest long-term impact on the way we view children. The "perfect child" mentality derives in part from the trend toward small families and a desire to maximize the potential of our children. It also reflects our overconfidence in technology. This chapter focuses attention on these implications of human genetic and reproductive technologies for children and families.

THE IMPACT OF REPRODUCTIVE TECHNOLOGIES ON CHILDREN

The literature is replete with references to the rights of women or couples to use reproductive technologies (*Harvard Law Review* 1985). The right to establish a family, the right to privacy in procreative matters, and the right to make intimate family decisions combine to guarantee significant ethical and legal support for prospective parents in the use of these technologies. The rights and needs of infertile couples or individuals who wish to have access to these innovations raise a responsive chord in U.S. society.

Conspicuously absent in most of the debate over reproductive technologies is analysis of the impact of these innovations on children—both as the direct products of the technologies and as concepts. First, what about the rights and needs of the child produced through reproductive mediating technology (TMR)? Certainly, the child is the person most affected by the decision to utilize TMR, but the child is not even a party to the decision. At the time of the decision, the resulting child is unable to make his or her point of view known. Although a case can be made that such a child would favor the decision of the parent(s) to use TMR, because otherwise he or she would have never existed, application of more advanced genetic interventions may weaken this argument. Although no child can consent to the circumstances of his or her birth, as Snowden et al. (1983) caution, we must remember that the desired outcome of TMR is the deliberate creation of a child. Therefore, "in making decisions and undertaking procedures to fulfill the wishes of the would-be parents it would be improper to forget that some child must live with the consequences of those decisions and procedures" (Snowden et al. 1983:25).

A second issue regarding the fate of children related to TMR revolves around the social value we place on the child. Until recently parents had children for a variety of personal reasons, but in the absence of the procreative technologies available today, they took responsibility for the children they bore. When fate dealt them a child with imperfections, largely they accepted it and coped as well as they could. Today, within the context of the expanding selection of intervention possibilities, many persons are no longer satisfied with a child viewed as less than the best. Even the average does not seem good enough for many parents. According to Klass (1989:45), "the search for a perfect baby is leading us further and further back into pregnancy," as the possibilities for earlier prenatal diagnosis multiply.

This desire for children who are "perfect" has significant long-term implications on our perceptions of children. As couples and singles limit their family to one or two children, their demand increases for technologies which they believe can guarantee that "perfect" child. According to many observers (see Bishop and Waldholz 1986) some young couples are now going to considerable lengths to ensure the birth of their perceived near-perfect child, including sex preselection. As more precise and effective genetic techniques emerge, pressures for access will intensify. Survey data indicate that many parents would consider termination of a pregnancy for even moderate defects in the unborn child, such as a heightened risk of early heart disease or criminal tendency. For instance, one survey (Keeton and Baskin 1985) found that 76 percent of the respondents would consider an abortion if their fetus was diagnosed as having any one of a range of serious disorders. Thirty-eight percent would consider an abortion of a fetus identified as having a heightened risk of early heart disease, muscular dystrophy, or blindness. Similarly, in a 1988 Gallup poll (*Hippocrates* 1988:40) 56 percent of the respondents agreed (34 percent disagreed) that abortion is justified when "Down's Syndrome or other major birth defects have been spotted by tests."

Many parents are likely not only to abort fetuses diagnosed as having problems, but also to use gene therapy to help them produce the child of their specifications. Keeton and Baskin (1985:287) found that 83 percent of their respondents would consider making genetic changes in their child for health reasons. Additionally, 11 percent would consider using genetic intervention to increase intelligence and 9 percent to enhance personality characteristics. Significantly, only 7 percent said they would not consider making genetic changes if it became possible. Recent evidence of parents demanding human growth hormone "therapy" for their healthy child, simply because they have been informed that the child would not be as tall as they desired, attests to the strength of this quest for the perfect child (Grumbach 1988).

As the success rates of TMRs heighten and become routinely used by infertile couples who desire their "own" child, the institution of adoption will be threatened. Although the supply of healthy Caucasian newborns is constricted in many locales, there are at present many adoptable older children and children with "special needs" that are not adopted. What will be their fate if we divert even more attention from their adoption as an option to childlessness? Permanent Families for Children and other organizations established to encourage adoption of such children will have a more difficult time placing them in a context where couples are convinced that new technologies are the answer to their infertility.

This emphasis on technological "perfection" raises questions concerning the purpose of children in this generation. It is not surprising that terms such as "quality control" over the reproductive process and children as "products" of particular techniques are commonplace. With the increased availability of sex and characteristic selection techniques, motivations for their application must be examined closely. There is a clear danger of viewing children as commodities, despite Andrews' (1986:201) claim that: "there is little evidence for the assertion that manipulating human reproduction will foster a dehumanizing attitude in society in general, causing us to look upon children as consumer goods." I argue that once the novelty of TMRs wears off and they become routine, the commodification of children will heighten. Survey data cited above, I believe, support this position. Although Andrews' (1986:201) claim that TMRs affect so few children as compared to divorce is certainly well taken and indicates that caution is needed in addressing these new technologies, the potential long-term impact of TMRs on the value of children cannot be underestimated.

In the least, these possible consequences of reproductive intervention dictate the urgency of substantial research regarding the social and psychological impact on the children. In our quest to achieve more control over the quality of our progeny, we have not committed equal resources to developing emotional and sociological profiles of the products of these technologies. The fact that most babies of AID are not told the circumstances of their birth (Rowland 1985), indicates a fear on the part of many people that such information could be damaging. Although it might be far more harmful not to reveal the truth, and research might affirm this, current behavior of these parents implies a fear of the truth. Even more harmful might be the emotional impact on the child who is the product of embryo lavage. How do the parents explain to a child that, as a five-day-old embryo, he or she was flushed from an anonymous genetic mother's uterus and transferred to the womb of his or her mother by a clinician in the laboratory? Or do they tell?

Furthermore, it is probable that the availability of technologies for prenatal diagnosis, genetic screening, and characteristic selection will heighten discrimination of children born with congenital or genetic disorders. Already, there is a clear danger that acceptance of selective abortion reduces tolerance for the living affected. Leon Kass (1976:317) expresses concern for those abnormals who are viewed as having escaped the "net of detection and abortion," as attitudes toward such individuals are "progressively eroded." In this atmosphere, affected individuals increasingly will be viewed as unfit to be alive, as second-class humans, at best, or as unnecessary persons who would not have been born if only someone had gotten to them in time. Parents are likely to resent such a child, especially if social pressures and stigma are directed against them. For Alexander Capron (1979:681), the recognition of an enforceable right to be born with a sound, normal mind and body would "open the door to judicially mediated genetic intervention of limitless dimensions." The choice of those affected is not between a healthy and unhealthy existence, but rather between an unhealthy existence and none at all.

Although Motulsky and Murray (1983:290) conclude that significant change in attitudes toward the living handicapped and their parents is not yet evident, "the potential of reducing the frequency of certain genetic diseases by selective abortion has raised the

question of possible discrimination against parents and patients
with diseases that could have been avoided with prenatal diagnosis."

For Stephen Stich (1983:9), the desire to help one's children
excel is a "powerful and widespread motivational force." With the
availability of techniques for genetically engineering traits that
convey a competitive advantage (such as increased intelligence,
memory, and longevity, as well as personality) parental demand to
maximize their progeny's chances will be substantial. Moreover,
those parents who are unable or unwilling to use these technologies
might find their offspring condemned to a second-class citizenry,
where what had been within the range of the normal gradually
slips into the domain of the subnormal (Stich 1983:10). Given our
litigious society, it would not be surprising to see children sue their
parents for failing to use available genetic enhancing technologies,
a failure which put them at a competitive disadvantage (see discussion of torts for wrongful life below).

Stich (1983) foresees even more drastic effects of human genetic
technology on human nature. In a society where prospective parents are able to choose from a library of genes to design their own
offspring, it is conceivable that not all people or all societies will
make the same choices. If different societies, or groups within
societies, systematically select for different traits over several generations, we could begin to see the genetic fragmentation of the
human species. At the extreme, divisions that separate cultural
groups might come to include genetic differences so profound that
members of the different groups would no longer be interfertile
(Stich 1983:10). Under such conditions, the common moral ground
that many observers assume all humans by their nature share,
despite other differences, would break down resulting in severe
repercussions across all societies. Although this scenario seems
unlikely, trends in our ability to intervene in the human genome
ought to cause us to contemplate how we wish to proceed.

Another danger of this quest for the perfect child through technology is that in the aggregate it might represent a eugenic mentality. Even if it can be argued to be in the interest of a particular
child to be a product of AID, IVF, SM, and so forth,

It is in the interest of children and families "in general" for the state
to foster a sense of security about them and to remove temptation by
not allowing sales of family members for money. (Field 1988:28)

Although this concern, I believe, is not enough to preclude the use of reproductive technologies, it must be introduced into any policy-making deliberations. In combination with the problem of com-modification of children that results from the commercialization of reproduction, the eugenic issue requires a more careful analysis of the consequences of the reproductive revolution. Although these concerns over a eugenic effect are certainly speculative at this stage, several current legal trends illustrate how insidious these consequences might be.

Torts for Wrongful Life

"By far the most unusual and troublesome set of liability issues that has thus far emerged from the intersection of law and human genetics" is the tort for "wrongful life" (Capron 1979:681). A tort for wrongful life is a suit brought on behalf of an affected infant, most commonly against a physician or other health professional who, it is alleged, negligently failed to inform the parents of the possibility of their producing a severely defective child, thereby preventing the parents from choosing to avoid its conception or birth. The unique aspect of such suits is the assumption that a life has evolved which should not have. If not for some negligence of the defendant, the child plaintiff would never have been born. Although the term "wrongful life" has been applied to a variety of situations, including those where parents are suing a third party for damages to the child (wrongful birth), it is more precise to limit wrongful life action to that brought solely by the affected *child*. Most recent suits for wrongful life have been brought on behalf of children with severe mental or physical defects asking for mone-tary damages to be awarded on the basis of the plaintiff's exis-tence, as compared to a state of nonexistence. In effect, the infant plaintiff claims that for him nonexistence would have been prefer-able to life and that he should be awarded damages for being forced to live that life.

Legal Precedents and Trends. Prior to the late 1970s, the courts unanimously refused to recognize the possibility of a cause of ac-tion for wrongful life. *Gleitman v. Cosgrove* (1967), in which the New Jersey Supreme Court declared that the preciousness of hu-man life, no matter how burdened, outweighs the need for recovery by the infant, set the precedent until well after *Roe v. Wade* (1973) altered public policy toward abortion. To award damages to the affected child would be counter to public policy, which views the right to life as inalienable in our society. This rejection of a wrongful life concept, however, changed with *Curlender v. Bio-Science Laboratories* (1980), in which a California appeals court agreed that a Tay-Sachs infant was entitled to seek recovery for alleged wrongful life. The court dismissed without discussion the central rationale for barring recovery in previous wrongful life cases since *Gleitman*—the value of nonexistence versus life with handicap—and focused attention instead on the resulting condition of the child.

> The reality of the "wrongful-life" concept is that such a plaintiff both exists and suffers, due to the negligence of others. It is neither necessary nor just to retreat into meditation on the mysteries of life. We need not be concerned with the fact that had defendants not been negligent, the plaintiff might not have come into existence at all. The certainty of genetic impairment is no longer a mystery. In addition a reverent appreciation of life compels recognition that the plaintiff, however impaired she may be, has come into existence as a living person with certain rights. (*Curlender* at 488)

In *Schroeder v. Perkel* (1981), a New Jersey court agreed with *Curlender* and allowed an infant plaintiff born with cystic fibrosis to collect for his "wrongful," "diminished" life. Moreover, in January 1983, a unanimous decision of the Supreme Court of Washington State in *Harbeson v. Parke-Davis* strongly approved the principle of wrongful life as well as wrongful birth. The court found that the parents have a right to prevent the birth of a defective child and that health care providers have a duty to impart to the parents material information about the likelihood of birth defects in their future children. The child born with such defects has a right to bring a wrongful life action against the health provider. According to the court, it would be illogical to permit parents, but not the child, to recover for the cost of the child's own medical care. Similarly, in a 1984 decision (*Procanik v. Cillo*), the New Jersey Supreme Court agreed with the Washington court and ruled that a congenitively defective child may maintain an action to recover at least the extraordinary medical expenses he or she will incur in his lifetime. Although the difficulty of determining how to measure damages for a claim that nonexistence is better than life in a defective condition remains a "vexing problem," according to the court, this does not prevent recovery of extraordinary medical expenses, which are predictable and certain.

Other recent decisions recognizing a cause of action for wrongful life against third parties are *Call v. Kerzirian* (1982) and *Graham v. Pima City* (1983). In *Call*, a California appeals court ruled that damages for extraordinary expenses for specialized teaching and training and special equipment that an unhealthy infant will need because of her defect are recoverable. In *Graham*, the Pima City Superior Court approved a settlement of $38,000 for a wrongful life action. Also see *Eisbrenner v. Stanley* (1981), where a physician's failure to diagnose rubella in a pregnant woman who subsequently gave birth to a deformed child served as a basis for a wrongful life claim.

Although these cases might demonstrate a trend in tort law, many courts continue to refuse to recognize wrongful life actions. In *Ellis v. Sherman* (1984), the Superior Court of Pennsylvania affirmed a lower court's refusal to recognize an infant's cause of action for wrongful life. This case involved the failure of an obstetrician to diagnose the manifestations of neurofibromatosis, a hereditary disorder which the father exhibited. Likewise, in *Alquijay v. St. Luke's-Roosevelt Hospital Center*, the New York County Supreme Court, Appellate Division, held that there is no cause of action on behalf of an infant to enable her to recover extraordinary expenses that would result of the disease after she reached her majority. In this case, an infant girl afflicted with Down's Syndrome was suing the hospitals whose personnel conducted amniocentesis which erroneously indicated the mother would give birth to a normal male child. The court reiterated its opposition on public policy grounds and concluded that recognition of such a cause of action would require legislation. Moreover, in *Di Natale v. Lieberman* (1982), the Michigan Appellate Court denied a cause of action for wrongful life because of the difficulty in assessing damages for being born, while in *Dorlin v. Providence Hospital* (1982), and *Nelson v. Krusen* (1982), the child's claim for wrongful life was rejected because the assessment of damages would be too speculative. The judicial landscape, then, continues to be eccentric and confusing.

A major development in wrongful life action since 1981 is the increased involvement of state legislatures. At least twelve legislatures have considered wrongful life causes of action. Of these, at least four have enacted measures limiting or prohibiting actions brought by, or on behalf of, infant plaintiffs for wrongful life. A 1982 Minnesota statute, for example, proscribes such tort actions, stating that: "No persons shall maintain a cause of action or receive an award of damages on behalf of himself based on the claim that but for the negligent conduct of another, he would have been aborted." A few states, including Idaho, have gone a step further and prohibited wrongful birth as well as wrongful life suits. This means that parents are unable to claim damages for the birth of an unhealthy child even if a physician fails to inform them of available prenatal tests that could have diagnosed the problem and given the parents the option of obtaining an abortion.

Although the motivation for such legislative action undoubtedly is complex, in several instances it has been overtly a product of anti-abortion sentiment. Right-to-life groups have argued successfully that the acceptance of wrongful life (and wrongful birth, in some cases) torts encourages abortion not only of those fetuses identified as defective but also of those fetuses that are marginal. Moreover, opponents of this cause of action assert that a legal atmosphere where wrongful life claims are recognized will encourage (coerce) health care providers to order diagnostic tests that are conducted only for "search and destroy" purposes to avoid liability. Advocacy groups for handicapped persons have also been critical of the use of technologies which are directed solely towards the end of selective abortion, instead of towards treatment of the handicap.

Social Implications of Torts for Wrongful Life. The concept of wrongful life vividly demonstrates the interaction among reproductive technology, social values, and the law. Decisions made in these cases both reflect the new knowledge offered by the technologies and influence the application of these technologies throughout society. The law not only is responsive to social values on quality-of-life matters, but also is a powerful force in shaping these values. As a result, wrongful life decisions have a heightened importance for defining the boundaries of responsibility for genetic disease within the dynamic and rapidly expanding context of technology.

The literature is replete with reference to the dangerous consequences of recognizing a cause of action for wrongful life. Oft-quoted is the statement in *Zepeda v. Zepeda* (1963) that the "legal implications of such a tort are vast, the social impact could be staggering." Some observers (Trotzig 1980:15) predict a "flood of litigation" and multimillion dollar settlements imposing an "intolerable burden" on the medical community, escalating maternity costs, and reducing services in some cases. Chapman (1979:34) notes a fear that "Down's Syndrome children from all over could come into court and sue were such an action recognized." Others dispute these claims and argue that relatively few children would be able to assert reasonably that they would have been better off not being born. Those in favor of awarding damages usually emphasize traditional tort functions of justice to the harmed, deterrence, and punishment.

If responses to other malpractice actions can be taken as examples, it appears reasonable to assume that many physicians and health professionals will react by practicing defensively. Although this is a desired goal of torts when it results in better care, wrongful life situations present a unique dilemma, since this response is manifested most clearly in heightened use of prenatal diagnosis and abortion of affected fetuses. As a result, judicial recognition of wrongful life actions might "induce physicians to abort all borderline fetuses," including those whose karyotypes or biochemical patterns are ambiguous or those whose prenatal diagnoses reveal minimal genetic defects (Friedman 1974:154). Moreover, physicians might be less prone to use heroic neonatal intensive care to save severely premature infants, for fear of later being sued for keeping them alive, though with damages.

Although a more realistic defense against negligence would appear to be full disclosure to the parents by the physician and referral to specialists who are more knowledgeable in genetics, it is likely that an atmosphere could develop which assumes that the most effective protection from wrongful life torts is to ensure that such infants are not born. Trotzig might be correct in anticipating this response from some physicians, but it seems improbable that wrongful life torts will become so pervasive as to dominate medical decision making. Such torts still require proof of duty, damage, negligence, and proximate cause, traditionally required by malpractice cases.

More crucial, however, is the potential impact of acceptance of the concept of wrongful life on perceptions by the public of those persons born with genetic or other congenital defects. Sorenson (1974:172) contends that the amount of prejudice now expressed toward mentally and physically disabled persons is already "generally more than that expressed toward various minority groups." If the courts recognize wrongful life, it is probable that these attitudes will be accentuated and social intolerance for the disabled will intensify because, it might be presumed, they should not have been born in light of the technologies available. It might also be feasible under such conditions for society to sue parents for the costs of maintaining such children in public institutions, although in the United States this would require substantial value altera- tions. Will insurance companies have an "out" if parents refuse to use routinely available technologies?

Although it is probable that a heightened discrimination of the genetically disabled will occur anyway as prenatal technologies are widely accepted, torts for wrongful life might strengthen the attitude that only "pristine pure health is tolerable." The danger of establishing arbitrary categories of individuals "rightfully" born and "wrongfully" born is obvious. "A cogent policy justification for the continued dismissal of wrongful life actions, is the possible societal acceptance of the belief that if the life of a genetically defective being is wrongful, then openly his death can be 'rightful'" (Friedman 1974:154). Ironically, what is viewed as "protecting the rights" of the plaintiff in a particular case might cumulatively result in degrading the rights of those affected by genetic disease as a group. As noted by Botkin (1988:1545), "children with disabil- ities will not be better served by the further development of the concept of life without value."

One extension of the concept of wrongful life that promises a severe impact on social values and on notions of responsibility is that situation where a damage claim is brought against the par- ents, charging their liability for their own child's birth under hand- icap. For instance, what liability do parents have if, given accurate advice from the physician regarding the risk of genetic disease, they disregard the advice and either fail to undergo prenatal diag- nosis or refuse to abort the abnormal fetus, resulting in a child with a genetic disorder? If a claim for damages against a physician can stand, can not a suit against the parents also succeed? In 1981, in response to this concern, the California legislature passed, and the governor signed, a bill stating that no cause of action arises against a parent of a child based upon the claim that the child should not have been conceived or, if conceived, should not have been allowed to have been born alive.

Until now, in cases of genetic disease, one has been able to argue that the parents could not be held accountable for circumstances beyond their control. The child's handicap is simply an unfortunate fate. As noted here, however, there is evidence that, given the state of human reproductive technology, the legal climate is moving toward sympathy for the affected child. Should such a practice become commonplace and children be awarded compensation for their genetic handicaps, society would find itself condoning a discriminate form of negative eugenics that ultimately could be applied to a wide range of conditions including intelligence, physical health, and emotional well-being. Capron (1980) suggests that the acceptance of such torts or similar actions by other "agencies of social control" might lead to "unprecedented eugenic totalitarianism."

What are the implications, if litigation by an infant plaintiff (most likely initiated by counsel representing his or her rights) is successful and he or she is awarded damages from the parents for birth with specific disabilities because the parents' "irresponsible" action had contributed to the disability? Had the parents given birth to a fetus known to be defective, part of their responsibility might be perceived as compensating the resulting child, even though the plaintiff would not exist if the parents made the opposite decision. One result would be that parental responsibility might evolve into a legal duty to refrain from having children under a variety of circumstances or to abort all defective fetuses. Many observers view this possibility with repugnance, but Shaw envisions beneficial results in this redefinition of parental responsibility:

> if the freedom to choose whether or not to have a child is limited by the threat of civil liability for having a child who is genetically defective, our posterity will be the beneficiaries. We will have decided that there is no "absolute right to reproduce" and that instead it is a "limited privilege" to contribute one's genetic heritage to future generations. (Shaw 1978:340)

What might appear to be a just and humane means of compensating children for damages suffered in specific cases, then, in reality might serve to redefine parental responsibility in procreation more generally. Torts for wrongful life have strong potential to encourage or coerce parents to reevaluate their value systems, which primarily assume the child to have limited rights vis-a-vis the parents. In addition to the individualist premise that each person has the "right" to be born free of defects to the maximum extent possible, such torts also include a societal dimension relating to responsibilities toward future generations. Both of these aspects might conflict directly with and limit the parents' procreation prerogatives. The eugenic implications of such lawsuits appear to be unplanned and simply a byproduct of the set of individual suits, but encouragement of such action by society might reflect an underlying predisposition to control procreation decisions and consciously limit parental discretion.

Although many courts continue to be unwilling to award damages based on "unavertable genetic diseases," the context is being altered substantially by broadened availability and knowledge of ever more sophisticated prenatal diagnostic and screening techniques. If the parents consciously reject prenatal diagnosis in a clear case of risk, refuse to participate in available carrier screening programs, or fail to use genetic therapy once that is feasible, and a handicapped child is born because of their action or lack of action, the child would appear to have reasonably strong cause of action once the wrongful life concept is accepted. Although the actual cause of the disability does not result directly from parental negligence, their failure to take prudent action to avoid the situation might be persuasive evidence against the parents.

Obviously, the merits of any case revolve around the certainty that such a disability could have been avoided through actions of the parents. As the state of human reproductive technology and the capacity to intervene at the gene level advance to provide effective means of alleviating fetal disorders, the parents might be expected to bear legal, as well as moral, responsibility for their actions in accepting or rejecting available technologies. In the absence of more direct compulsory eugenic legislation, torts for wrongful life serve as one means by which society defines "responsible" and "irresponsible" procreation decisions. If the courts recognize the rights of progeny to sue their parents for damages, this would represent a strong, though indirect, mandate to parents predisposed against human intervention technologies to utilize them. By allowing compensation to affected children through wrongful life torts, society, as reflected in its courts, would put its mark of disapproval on such parental actions.

Torts for wrongful life certainly do not compare in poignancy to direct eugenic efforts, such as compulsory sterilization, and most probably can be justified on other grounds. They could, however, represent an effective social pressure or "unwritten social mandate" to conform to societal standards. Because they are less obviously a social sanction on childbearing decisions than other eugenic techniques and in fact are presented as a means of protecting the "rights" of the affected child, torts for wrongful life provide an even greater challenge for those concerned with life and death issues than the more obvious forms of eugenics. Their very subtlety obscures broader implications for the value system.

REPRODUCTIVE TECHNOLOGIES AND THE STATUS OF WOMEN

Next to the children who are products of genetic and reproductive technologies, the most affected group in society is women. As noted earlier, the conventional definition of motherhood is undergoing rapid transformation as technology intervenes and cleaves the procreative process. As a result:

> Noncoital reproductive techniques pose a challenge to feminist analysis. They offer new possibilities for personal choice at the same time as they exacerbate possibilities for exploiting some women or reinforce societal attitudes concerning the imperative of biological parenthood. (Office of Technology Assessment 1988:326)

Woliver (1989:43) contends that reproductive technologies often contain hidden policy implications—"they increase medical intervention in women's lives, diminishing women's power over their bodies and babies."

Arditti (1985:582) points out that splitting motherhood into bits and pieces weakens women's claim to maternity. The integrity of motherhood disappears when one woman can donate the egg, one can carry the fetus to term, and a third raises the child. According to Arditti (1985:582), "in this dismemberment of maternity, women may lose one of our few (potential) sources of power." Mies is more vehement in her indictment of reproductive technologies as inherently sexist:

> Sexist biases permeate the new reproductive technologies and genetic engineering at all levels. In general they imply that motherhood, the capacity of women to bring forth children, is changed from a creative process, in which woman cooperated with her body as an active human being, to an industrial production process. In this process, not only is the symbiosis of mother and child disrupted, but the whole process is rationalized, objectified, planned and controlled by medical experts. More than ever before the woman is objectified and made passive. (1987:332)

Furthermore, because the woman is no longer one whole object, but rather a series of objects that can be isolated, examined, recombined, sold, hired, or simply thrown away, the integrity of the woman as a human person is destroyed (Mies 1988:332).

Although individual women might benefit from reproductive technologies, the cumulative effect on women might be to jeopardize their freedom. According to Hubbard (1982:210), when "choices" become available to women, they all too rapidly become compulsions to "choose" the alternative endorsed by society. For Petchesky (1980:685):

> The "right to choose" means very little when women are powerless. . .women make their own reproductive choices, but they do not make them just as they please; they do not make them under conditions which they themselves create but under social conditions and constraints which they, as mere individuals, are powerless to change.

Furthermore, these technologies contribute to a medicalization of reproduction that threatens the freedom and dignity of women in general. By requiring third party involvement and dependence on medical technique, TMRs force the woman to surrender control over procreation. Elsewhere, Hubbard (1985:567) decries the practice of making every pregnancy a medical event, and sees it as a result of the economic incentives for physicians to stimulate a new need for their services during pregnancy, in light of declining birth rates and increasing interests in midwives and home birth. Rothman (1986:114) adds that the new images of the fetus resulting from prenatal technologies are making us aware of the "unborn" as people, "but they do so at the cost of making transparent the mother." Furthermore, a "diagnostic technology that pronounces judgments halfway through the pregnancy makes extraordinary demands on women to separate themselves from the fetus within."

One example of the medicalization of reproduction centers on the use of AID. The woman is cast in the role of a patient upon which treatment is given even though no medical indication on her part is exhibited. If anything, her spouse, who is uninvolved in the procedure other than to give his consent, is the patient in absentia. At best, the medical setting functions to legitimize AID for the woman and for society. Ironically, research into male infertility might have a higher priority if AID were not so easy, and—as some feminists argue—done to the woman (Corea 1985). In a growing number of cases, AID is carried out because the husband had earlier undergone sterilization voluntarily, only to change his mind as circumstances changed.

Similarly, IVF increasingly is being used on healthy, fertile women to enable them to have children fathered by their infertile male partners. Because in vitro fertilization requires only a small proportion of viable sperm as compared to natural fertilization, men with very low sperm counts (functionally infertile for uterine fertilization) might father a child if their spouse undergoes IVF. This particular application of IVF again illustrates that the "choices" opened up to women by TMRs many times are illusory.

Feminists rightly argue that women bear most of the risks of any reproductive research and technological application. According to Oakley (1984:24) the history of human reproduction has been, in large measure, the saga of control of women, their fertility and fecundity, by society. This control, whether self imposed or inflicted by others in a given society, has resulted in a significant loss of freedom to women and their exclusion from many activities including intellectual creativity, waged work, and training for self-support. Women, it is argued, have been held hostage to the reproductive needs of society throughout history, and the new reproductive technologies in many ways reinforce this condition.

To some extent, the fact that women bear the risks of reproductive technology is explained by their biologically central role in pregnancy. There seems, nevertheless, to be a bias in favor of research that leads to intervention in women, not men, and thereby places them at risk. Many feminists assert that the problem is exacerbated because the majority of researchers and clinicians are male (Corea 1985a). Rowland (1985a:544), for instance, argues:

> We are discussing here the making of reputations for male medical researchers, and the making of money for male-owned and controlled companies. Women-controlled use of this technology is not part of the scenario envisaged by those who make and own these processes.

Once again, it is argued (see Rothschild 1983) that women are being excluded from the debate in society about human reproduction. Although they are most affected by these technologies, women are virtually absent from the legal, scientific, and governmental bodies which design the research, development, and delivery of the technologies.

For Arditti (1985:581), there is a major difference between a woman who would be a surrogate for a friend and the situation where lawyers and gynecologists are forming companies "for the purpose of selling women's reproductive powers to strangers." The skepticism of feminists toward TMRs is certainly warranted, although there is disagreement even among feminists as to the best policy to surmount the problems.

There is little doubt that the status of women is intimately related to human genetic and reproductive technologies. Technology is never neutral—it both reflects and shapes social values. Because of women's critical biological role as the bearers of children, any technologies that deal with reproduction affect their social role directly. Moreover, because these technologies focus on the role of women as mothers, they could lead to diminution of other roles. Feminists argue that too much emphasis is already placed on women as mothers only in this society. Infertility indicates for many women a barren and useless life. Reproductive technologies reinforce this view. According to Rowland, women must reevaluate this social overstatement of the role of motherhood. "The catchcry but women want it has been sounded over and over again by the medical profession to justify continuing medical advances in this field. Women need to reevaluate just what it is they want and question this justification for turning women into living laboratories" (New Zealand 1986:39).

Commercialization of human reproduction, especially raises critical issues for women. On the one hand, this trend promises to make these techniques more widely available to women who want them. They offer women choices that were until recently unthinkable. Just as commercialization easily leads to commodification of children, it also leads to a value context where gametes, embryos, and women are viewed as commodities to be "banked, bought, sold, and rented as a means to procreation" (OTA 1988:327). Surrogate motherhood, especially, raises the issue of potential exploitation of women by entrepreneurs of the SM industry. For Field (1988:27), having a baby is such a personal event that it should be kept out of the marketplace. "A system of agencies reaping profits by arranging for surrogate mothers and of surrogate mothers earning substantial fees by having babies commercializes childbearing to the detriment of us all." She decries the commodification of women and their experience in childbearing, and points out the danger of objectifying the woman by talk of rent-a-womb or the use of a surrogate uterus (Field 1988:29). On the other hand, the prohibition of SM contracts might be construed as patronizing to women and a threat to their rights—another protectionist ploy of policy makers.

Also, while prenatal diagnosis, genetic screening, gene therapy, sex preselection, and so forth, expand options and will largely be used by women, as argued earlier, they carry a causal logic that could label as socially irresponsible women who fail to make use of them under certain circumstances. As Hubbard (1985:567) cogently states: "The point is that once such a test is available and a woman decides not to use it, if her baby is born with a disability that could have been diagnosed, it is no longer an act of fate but has become her fault." Meis (1988:334) adds that the emphasis on quality control means for most women a loss of confidence in their own bodies and their childbearing competence. She argues that the social pressure on women to produce perfect children is already enormous today.

Although the technologies that allow for the conscious design of children do not necessarily result in the denigration of the role of women or the restriction of their reproductive rights, within the context of a social value system sympathetic to that end, the danger clearly exists. A full policy assessment of these technologies, therefore, requires close attention to their cumulative impact on women as well as to women's actual experiences as reproductive beings (Overall 1987). This, again, requires a widened commitment of policy makers to fund extensive behavioral research on women who are parties to these reproductive applications or who are contemplating using these services.

REPRODUCTIVE TECHNOLOGIES AND THE FAMILY

Reproductive technologies are often touted as family enhancing innovations (U.S. Congress 1987b), and to the extent that they allow some couples to have children who otherwise could not, they are. When one looks beyond the specifics of individual cases to the broader, long-term implications on social values regarding the family, the situation becomes more nebulous. These technologies are controversial in large part because they challenge deeply held values concerning the family and the relationships among its members. They deliberately separate reproduction from the human body and bring third parties into the relationship as facilitators of the technological process, thus compromising the "deeply held conviction that matters pertaining to reproduction are and should be matters of private concern" (King 1986:113). As torts for wrongful life illustrate, decisions made in specific cases to compensate a harm cumulatively can alter family relationships and pit parents against child. Similarly, the availability of prenatal diagnosis, gene therapy, and fetal surgery can lead to a causal logic that labels as irresponsible parental decisions not to take advantage of them. As noted earlier, one set of parents' right to use these technologies could be another set of parents' duty once the techniques become socially accepted.

Collaborative Conception

One area where there is a clear interaction between advances in reproductive mediating technologies and genetic diagnosis, which has an impact on familial decision-making, centers on parental responsibility for use of the former for individuals identified as carriers of a genetic disease or susceptibility. Is there a duty of such parents to forego their right to reproduction, either by refraining from procreation or using collaborative conception technologies such as AI or embryo transfer so as not to transmit the deleterious genes to their offspring? If there is such a duty, where are the lines to be drawn: a genetic disease like Huntington's or sickle-cell anemia; a heightened risk for manic depression or alcoholism; or susceptibility to early heart disease? Purdy (1978:26), for instance, contends "it is wrong to reproduce when we know there is a high risk of transmitting a serious disease or defect."

Here again a causal logic is triggered. Until recently, the only option for averting the birth of the affected child was to refrain from having children, perhaps to adopt. With the advent of prenatal tests for certain recessive diseases, where the chance of having an affected child is 25 percent if both parents are carriers, another technological option was opened. For each pregnancy they could make use of the appropriate prenatal test to determine the status of the fetus. If the fetus did not have the disease they could carry it to term. If the test was positive they could exercise their constitutional right to an abortion or carry it to term with that knowledge, if they so chose. For many persons, particularly those opposed to abortion, this situation was untenable, because instead of treating the disease the life of the fetus with the disease was terminated. Of course, developments in gene therapy might alleviate this problem by permitting treatment of the affected fetus, but gene therapy of this form is yet in the realm of future hope.

With the development and increasing social acceptance of TMRs in the last decade, however, a new alternative is emerging. Instead of taking the chance of having an affected child or using prenatal diagnosis to allow informed selective abortion, a couple can now make use of collaborative conception by using the genetic material of nonaffected donors (assuming that donors of germ materials have been genetically screened). Now, for instance, if the husband of a couple is identified through DNA tests as carrying the dominant gene for Huntington's disease, the wife can undergo AID. If they are both identified as carriers of a deleterious gene, they can avert the conception of the one-of-four-affected child by using donor sperm, ova, or embryos.

Collaborative conception, thus, can be viewed as opening up the couple's options and giving them the means of having a family where they otherwise would have chosen not to. If any social coercion is used, however, no matter how subtle, it can threaten the right of couples to make intimate family decisions. At the least, collaborative conception brings third parties into the procreative equation, confuses traditional relationships within the family structure, and necessitates a careful reevaluation of the concept of family.

Although the popular media have tended to emphasize the up side of TMRs—with a multitude of pictures of the healthy, happy babies and blissful parents—the *Baby M* case dramatically demonstrated that both TMR children and parents can suffer. Whatever the final arrangements for custody and visitation of Melissa the courts determine, she is in for a confusing childhood at best. Although one can argue that she will face no more problems than other children caught in the middle of highly publicized custody battles, her plight is the direct result of an explicit intention to use technology to produce a child. She and other children of TMRs are the products of technologies that permit the deliberate separation of the biological and social parenting prior to fertilization. Although many children of TMR will not face this magnitude of publicity, the result is not always the happy ending often presented in magazine articles on TMRs and families.

Another consideration in TMRs is the potential adverse impact on other children in the family. How, for instance, did Mary Beth Whitehead's other children view her actions? As argued by Field

(1988:33), the picture of a mother handing over her child in exchange for money does not fit with traditional notions of parenthood. Although there is no data, one can surmise that the older children which many surrogate mothers have must be emotionally harmed. How does the SM explain giving away or selling their sibling and how can she make them believe that they do not have a similar price tag? Similarly, a child whose potential sibling's life is terminated prenatally for genetic or parental preference reasons must experience some psychological trauma. For these reasons, the use of RMTs should be proceeded by comprehensive family counseling of all members, including other children.

The New Extended Families

As noted earlier, reproductive technologies have revolutionized the definitions of motherhood and fatherhood by dividing the procreative process into discrete stages, each potentially performed by different persons. By doing so, TMRs allow many new combinations of parenthood, resulting in a new form of extended family comprised of multiple mothers or fathers and novel forms of relationships. Melissa Stern, for instance, has two mothers and possibly two fathers of some type (Dr. Stern and Mr. Gould, Mary Beth Whitehead's current husband). But what relationship, if any, does Richard Whitehead (Mary Beth's husband at the time she carried Melissa to term) have to Melissa? What relationship will Melissa have with her half-siblings? Who are her grandparents, and do they have any rights or responsibilities? What is her family history, or is concept no longer meaningful in defining a family? In many less acrimonious cases, the SM literally has moved in with the couple during her pregnancy and then becomes and "aunt" to the child and its siblings. Who are the grandparents of an SM baby and how much should the child be told of his or her real roots? The long-term psychological implications of such confusing arrangements for the child are yet to be determined. According to the OTA (1988:209), the opinion of experts varies as to the extent to which the genetic, gestational, and social functions of parenthood can be separated while still preserving the welfare of both the parents and children.

Finally, TMRs raise the issue of family bonding, a subject which has received considerable attention of late. Bonding between the infant and an adult is viewed as a prerequisite to the psychological and physical growth of the child. Furthermore, it sustains the abilities of the parents to nurture the child (OTA 1988:209). Which of the parents (genetic, gestational, social) has the right to form the parent-child bond? Because there is considerable evidence that mother-child bonding begins before birth, are there any circumstances where the gestational mother (i.e., surrogate mother) should be denied custody? Does the use of AID or SM to explicitly create a single-parent family violate a child's claim to bond with both a mother and a father, or is a father-child bonding insignificant?

TMRs have important ramifications on how parent-child bonding takes place and for possible new variations in the developing identities of children. If such bonding does have important psychological benefits for parents and is essential to the developing personalities of the product children, then considerably more research of the psychological impact of TMR on parents and, especially, the children is crucial at this stage, before use of the techniques becomes routine. To date, with all of the attention focused on these remarkable and revolutionary technologies, little effort has been directed to this dimension. If it turns out that the children of AID, SM, IVF, and the growing array of TMRs are emotionally scarred or harmed, this should be known before large numbers of desperate couples use such techniques. No matter how some persons attempt to reduce procreation to a technological process, we must eventually face the psychological impact on all parties to the process. We have much to gain and little to lose by slowing down the proliferation of reproductive services until that time when we have a better understanding of their impact on all members of the family.

Nontraditional Family Structures

Despite their introduction of collaborative conception and, thus, a confusion of family roles, the most extensive impact of RMTs on family structure promises to be their encouragement of single parent households and nontraditional parental combinations. RMTs have increased the options available to individuals who desire to create a family without traditional marriage ties. Reports of the use of surrogate mothers by wealthy single men who wish to have a child but without long-term legal responsibilities to a woman have been made (Keane and Breo 1981). More common are the increasingly vocal demands by lesbian women for access to AID for the purpose of procreation without intercourse. Kern and Ridolfi (1982:252) report that the use of AID as a means of parenthood for single women and lesbian couples is gaining popularity. One article (*Harvard Law Review* 1985:671) reports that at least 1500 unmarried women a year in the U.S. are artificially inseminated despite the difficulty of gaining access to AID services.

According to Snowden et al. (1983:13), once a stable marriage is no longer a precondition for AID, then the social and psychological implications for babies born in households where no males are present must be seriously considered. Although this is "not to say that lesbian couples or cohabiting women should be denied the right to have a baby by AID, but to point out need for rules within which the service is to be provided if the practice is not to change the basis of social organization—the family." One case in California is indicative of the confusion over parental roles that can follow use of RMTs. Two lesbian women wanted to have a baby. To do so, they obtained sperm which one of the two women artificially inseminated with a turkey baster into the uterus of the second. In a custody battle following breakup of the couple several years later, the first woman argued that she in fact was the "father" since she physically inseminated the "mother." Moreover, she argued it was their mutual intention that they share the parental roles. In this instance, the case was dismissed, but it does point out the problems with traditional family role definitions.

Reproductive technologies promise to revolutionize the family structure even more if the demands of some transsexual groups are ultimately met. These persons are genetic males who have undergone hormonal and surgical treatment to become females. Increasingly, some of these individuals are demanding more government funding of research into male procreation and rapid development of applications so that they can experience "womanhood to its fullest." As noted earlier, male procreation is likely to be possible in the near future. If transsexual women have access, it seems unlikely that other men who desire to experience "motherhood" will be denied it. The implications of this technique for family structure is staggering.

Equally revolutionary possibilities will exist should egg fusion research be successful and applicable to humans. In that event, two lesbian women could have "their" child using one egg from each woman, and so eliminate the need for any male contribution (and any chance of having a male child). In this case, the child would have two genetic mothers and no genetic father. An extension of this technique using both eggs from the same woman would give the girl one genetic mother and no genetic father. The heightened possibility of genetic disease in this case (since all the genes come from one person) should negate this application, but such a prohibition might have difficulty withstanding a constitutional challenge.

Although the small number of children conceived to single parents via RMT pales in comparison to the overall number of children now raised by single parents, these practices raise unique questions. Despite a trend toward single parent adoption in the U.S., the societal consequences of individuals conceiving with the explicit intention of raising a child alone must be analyzed. It is unlikely that access to these technologies by single parents, even transsexuals, could be prohibited without serious challenges on constitutional grounds (*Harvard Law Review* 1985). Kern and Ridolfi (1982:253), for instance, contend that single women's rights to be parents through AID are protected by the Fourteenth Amendment. They conclude

> However desirable the idealized nuclear family is to the majority, promotion of this ideal constitutes an insufficient justification for the state's suppression of alternative forms of intimate association, absent some showing of independent harm resulting from these alternatives. (252)

Similarly, the OTA (1988a:222) concludes:

> Nontraditional families—whether they consist of single parent and child, same-sex parents and child, or multiple parents. . .—provide emotional satisfaction and expression of personal identity in the same fashion as more traditional marital unions. Logically, then, this reasoning would extend the freedom of association and the freedom to procreate in any family form.

It goes on to state, however, that the difficulty of reconciling this reasoning with that which continues to support state authority to prohibit certain forms of sexual activity makes it "impossible to predict with certainty the Supreme Court's likely reaction to an assertion that nontraditional family privacy supports a right to procreate that extends to the use of noncoital reproductive techniques."

CONCLUSIONS: THE SOCIAL COSTS OF
DESIGNING OUR CHILDREN

Any technologies as powerful as the emerging human genetic and reproductive innovations are bound to disrupt traditional social structures. If their use is limited to a small proportion of the population, these changes are likely to be manageable, despite their impact on individual children and parents. If, however, use of the techniques becomes widespread or if they are routinely used in certain situations (e.g., prenatal diagnosis for women over age 35), they are likely to have severe repercussions. Also, the very availability of these technologies might produce a social climate in which refusal to accede to them will be viewed as irresponsible behavior. Under such circumstances, social pressure will compel use of the technologies which are now largely construed as expanding procreative choice.

Therefore, before we move too far into the era of designer children, we must rationally assess the implications for children, women, and the family. This requires an intensified agenda of behavioral research which includes in-depth follow up studies of families created through TMR. To what extent are the problems discussed here genuine and how widespread are they? Perhaps we will find that the dangers are overestimated, that TMR families as a whole are stronger than traditional ones. If that is the case, then we can with conviction and confidence support extension of TMRs. If these concerns are confirmed, however, policies to regulate these technologies are warranted on that ground. I argue that the potential harms to children, women, and families are severe enough to put the burden of proof on those who argue that TMRs are family-building interventions (U.S. Congress 1987b). It is critical at this juncture that the human costs of human reproductive intervention be carefully evaluated in light of their revolutionary impact on the most fundamental social values and structures. Along with commercialization and the inclusion of third parties in procreation, the long-term impact on the way we, as a society, view children and women demonstrates how essential it is to frame any public policy in light of these issues. At many levels, these technologies call for government involvement, despite the difficulties such activities raise. With this theme in mind, chapter 5 analyzes the current policy status in the United States and, chapter 6 describes policy developments in other countries.

CHAPTER FIVE

Current Regulatory Efforts: Public and Private

*I*N THE continuing absence of anything approaching a national
policy for regulation of reproductive technologies in the United
States, efforts to deal with their social impact currently are an
amalgam of largely uncoordinated private and public action. In
recent years, there have been major attempts at self-regulation of
particular applications by national associations such as the American Fertility Society and the American Association of Tissue Banks.
As illustrated by novel torts for wrongful life and wrongful birth
and difficult applications of existing case law (e.g., surrogate custody), the courts have emerged as active participants in setting
policy. Finally, in part spurred by such highly publicized court
cases as *Baby M*, state legislatures have begun to be more actively
involved in these issues.

To date, however, much of this action—both private and public

—has been reactive in nature, not anticipatory. Often the response has been a highly emotional one, as one technique comes quickly into the public limelight until replaced by attention to yet another technique and its attendant challenges to basic values. As a result, there has been very little in-depth analysis of the broader issues of this reproductive revolution and of the cumulative social impacts of this growing arsenal of human genetic and reproductive technologies. As Patricia King (1986:132) cogently states:

> the law clearly has not addressed most of the issues raised by the new reproductive technologies, and, where it has attempted to do so in the United States with respect to artificial insemination, the efforts have been inadequate. In the United States, the remaining reproductive technologies are virtually unregulated; the regulation that exists is basically the result of inadvertent coverage of other areas such as abortion or fetal research legislation.

This chapter reviews the current state of these disparate attempts to manage these powerful technologies of human reproduction. It concludes that these fragmentary, haphazard, and often inconsistent actions should be replaced at the least by coordinated national guidelines, if not regulations.

STATE GOVERNMENT INVOLVEMENT IN REPRODUCTION

Under the U.S. Constitution, the state legislatures, not Congress, are responsible for framing health policy. Congressional action, therefore, is usually a response to existing state legislation and serves primarily to establish minimum national standards and/or provide federal funds to encourage state action of a particular type. Federal court decisions (i.e., *Roe v. Wade*) also have been made in reaction to state statutes, either declaring specific legislation unconstitutional or liberalizing or standardizing state action. Although the role of the federal government on health policy vis-a-vis the states has expanded, especially since adoption of the Medicare/Medicaid programs in the mid-1960s, most initiation of policy continues to be made within the fifty states.

Under their authority to protect the public health, safety, and morals of the citizenry, states also retain the power to regulate familial relations, including marriage, divorce, adoption, and marital duties. Unless the federal government negates state law on constitutional grounds as it did with Texas' abortion law in *Roe*, it is the states which traditionally make laws most relevant to reproduction.

> Accordingly, the states have the authority to regulate noncoital reproductive techniques directly in a variety of ways. . . . The state's inherent powers to protect patients, research subjects, and perhaps even embryos are broad and provide many avenues for regulation. (OTA 1988:172)

Most relevant are the state's authority to license health care personnel and facilities, regulate medical malpractice litigation, place restrictions on the sale of embryos, and enact criminal statutes concerning activities deemed dangerous to public health, safety, or welfare.

In addition, contracts are generally regulated by each state, resulting in different degrees of enforceability of a contract type from state to state. Contracts to arrange for a surrogate mother, for instance, are subject to state law as are contracts between the producers and consumers of other reproductive technologies.

There are two main routes to state control: legislative statutes and common law. Statutes take precedence over common or judge-made law. In the absence of legislative action, however, common law becomes a crucial policy-making agent. In many states, non-consensual sterilization, torts for wrongful life, and the legal status of an AID child, among many other reproduction-related policies are based in common, not statutory, law. In some instances, state legislatures have acted to void precedents set by common law. In such cases, the statute is a direct response to the court action which the legislature views as contrary to its interpretation of public policy. As noted earlier, in the majority of states, most matters concerning human reproductive intervention are currently centered in common law. This situation, however, is bound to change as these issues become more salient and politically explosive.

The Legal Context of AID

Despite the widespread use of AID during the last three decades, legal questions abound. Because the children resulting from AID are not the complete biological offspring of the parents, the legitimacy of AID progeny has been frequently questioned, often in estate or divorce proceedings. The courts have been asked to decide if the husband, although not the biological father, is responsible for child support payments or, conversely, entitled to child visitation privileges. As is usual in a new area of law, court decisions have been inconsistent. In *Strnad v Strnad* (1948), a New York superior court held that an AID child was legitimate if the husband consented prior to the procedure. Under such circumstances, the court granted him the same rights as a natural father following divorce. Although most decisions have affirmed *Strnad*, some have not. In *Doornbos v Doornbos* (1954), for instance, an Illinois county court held that an AID child born to a married couple was conceived out of wedlock and was, therefore, illegitimate. After a series of court cases in California in which an AID child was declared illegitimate, a state appellate court held that the term "father" could not be restricted to its biological sense (*People v. Sorenson*, 1968). The court ruled that "the determinative factor is whether the legal relationship of the father and child exists" and concluded that consent of the father prior to AID was both legally binding and irreversible.

In addition to lingering questions concerning the status of the child and the husband, the rights and responsibilities of sperm donors have yet to be clarified in many jurisdictions. Can the donor secure access to files in order to locate his progeny? Does he have any control over who receives his sperm? Contrariwise, is there any risk the court will assign him paternal duties? In *C.M. v C.C.* (1979), the court addressed the question of donor rights in a case where the mother knew the donor and inseminated herself without presence of a third party. After the baby's birth, C.M. sought visitation privileges over the objections of C.C. The court ruled in favor of C.M, acknowledged him as the natural father, and granted him the privileges as well as responsibilities of fatherhood. This case illustrates the dangers of nonanonymous AID for the parties involved, but it cannot be viewed as a precedent for the vast majority of third-party or professionally mediated AID.

While the courts continued to grapple with the legal status of the child, the husband, and the donor, in the late 1960s many state legislatures became involved and largely clarified the situation in their states. At present, 30 states have passed statutes designed to clarify the paternity of a child conceived through AID (table 5.1). In all cases, they legitimize the AID child by providing that the sperm recipient and her husband are the legal parents if the husband consented prior to the procedure. Eleven of these statutes refer only to married women, thus leaving single women's use of AID in a legal limbo. The husband who gives consent, therefore, is the same under law as the natural father. These laws were largely

TABLE 5.1. Selected Provisions of State AID Statutes

State	Physician Must Inseminate	Refers only to Married Women	Mentions Husband Consent	Legitimizes Offspring	Requires Record-keeping
Alabama	x	x	x	x	x
Alaska		x	x	x	
Arkansas	x	x	x	x	
California	x		x	x	x
Colorado	x			x	
Connecticut	x		x	x	x
Florida			x	x	
Georgia	x			x	
Idaho	x		x	x	x
Illinois	x		x	x	
Kansas			x	x	x
Louisiana				x	
Maryland		x	x	x	
Michigan		x	x	x	
Minnesota	x			x	
Montana	x	x	x	x	x
Nevada	x	x	x	x	x
New Jersey	x			x	
New Mexico	x		x	x	x
New York	x	x	x	x	
North Carolina			x	x	
Ohio	x		x	x	x
Oklahoma	x		x	x	x
Oregon	x		x	x	x
Tennessee		x	x	x	
Texas		x	x	x	
Virginia	x	x	x	x	
Washington	x		x	x	x
Wisconsin	x		x	x	x
Wyoming	x		x	x	x

SOURCE: Adapted from OTA 1988a:243.

attempts to deal statutorily with custody suits that arose when the parents of AID children divorced. A contributing factor was the recognized need of protecting sperm donors from paternity suits.

Although these statutes do not make distinctions on the basis of method of AID, they seem to assume that it is done via anonymous donor through a professional service or physician. The status of the children of third-party-arranged, and especially AID with a known donor, such as in *C.M. v C.C.*, might be less certain, depending on the immediate context within which it was accomplished. For the vast majority of AID children in 30 states, however, these statutes have the merit of giving them legitimacy. The disadvantage is that the procedure of treating the husband as the natural father conceals the truth from the child. The advantage to the husband and wife is that they are clearly the legal parents. Overall, the sperm donor is protected by law from bearing any paternal responsibilities to the children conceived with his sperm. This consideration is critical for guaranteeing an adequate supply of willing sperm donors. Although the legal landscape of AID has been clarified by these statutes, almost half of the states have yet to address the issue. Their silence leaves the status of AID unresolved and dependent either upon case-by-case adjudication or shrouded by secrecy.

Some states continue to use the genetic link as the determining factor of parenthood, thereby forcing the husband to adopt the child in order to establish legal fatherhood. Without doubt, the consent-based approach for identification of the parents of a child is more sensible and reasonable than the genetic-based approach (Rosettenstein 1981). The child's parents in this case are those persons who want the child and have indicated their intention to raise the child. Despite a continued ambiguity over its status in some states, and the occasional lawsuits most commonly emerging from divorce custody hearings where the wife challenges the husband's claim to paternity of the child, after several decades AID largely is accepted as a legitimate method of aided reproduction that falls within the confines of a couple's right to privacy.

Although the debate over legitimacy of AID children appears to have been resolved in those states which have produced legislation, concern now has shifted toward criteria for donor selection. Curie-Cohen et al. (1979) in a survey of 379 practitioners of AID found a general lack of standards in donor selection, inadequate genetic screening of prospective donors, and a failure to keep adequate permanent records on donors. They also suggest that frequently the process places the interests of the physician and donor above that of the child. In part a response to the Curie-Cohen study, Oregon in 1981, passed a law providing that donors not knowingly have a genetic or venereal disease (Ore. Rev. Stat. sec. 109. 239). Idaho, too, makes it a violation of the Code (secs. 34–5401 to 39–5408, 1985) for a man who knowingly has a genetic or venereal disease to be a donor. Ohio requires, in addition to a full physical examination and genetic history, genetic screening of all AID donors. Only New Mexico limits the number of offspring per donor, even though this is recommended practice. Furthermore, twenty-one states require that AID be performed only by a licensed physician, presumably to assure at least some donor screening. The Georgia AI statute (Ga. Code Ann. sec. 74–101.1, 1973), for instance, provides that licensed physicians and surgeons are the only persons authorized to perform AI upon any female. Any other person who attempts or actually administers or performs AI upon any female human being is guilty of felony, with threat of punishment by imprisonment for not less than one year nor more than five years. Actually, the performance of AI by anyone not licensed to practice medicine, even in the absence of an explicit penalty, may constitute the unauthorized practice of medicine (Shaman 1980).

Other state legislation addresses the problem of inadequate record-keeping in AID transactions uncovered by Curie-Cohen. Fourteen states now require that records about the donor be kept sealed, and opened only by court order. Although these statutes probably discourage some potential sperm donors, they serve to protect the interests of AID children by allowing for the possibility of identifying paternity in order to diagnose heredity traits that might be linked to genetic disease.

Although sperm banks have been in existence for three decades and are obviously of legal and ethical concern, they are virtually unregulated (King 1986:129). Most of the current state statutes make no reference to cryobanks and those few which do make no effort to regulate them. The expansion of cryobanks and their increasing centrality to RMT requires a close analysis of how best to monitor their activities and guarantee consumer protection.

The Legal Context of IVF

Although IVF is now used in at least 190 clinics nationwide, little statutory regulation of it exists. In fact, only two states explicitly address therapeutic IVF. In 1982, Pennsylvania enacted the first

IVF statute (figure 5.1). Although the statute does nothing to impede the practice of IVF, the record-keeping and reporting provisions do allow the state to monitor IVF. In 1986, Louisiana enacted a statute that restricts practice of IVF to those facilities that comply with the guidelines of the American Fertility Society or the American College of Obstetricians and Gynecologists (details later in chapter). Several other states have laws that mention IVF but do not address its regulation. Kentucky addresses IVF in its adoption statutes only to state that nothing in the law prohibiting adoption in certain circumstances prohibits IVF. Illinois' fetal research law specifies that it is not intended to prohibit the "performance of IVF," while the New Mexico statute states that clinical uses of IVF are not covered by research regulations.

The recency of IVF and embryo transfer, as compared to AID, therefore, is reflected in a considerably less developed legislatory landscape. Many of the current laws only indirectly affect IVF or

---

FIGURE 5.1. Pennsylvania IVF Statute

In vitro fertilization—All persons conducting, or experimenting in, in vitro fertilization shall file quarterly reports with the department, which shall be available for public inspection and copying, containing the following information:

1. Names of all persons conducting or assisting in the fertilization or experimentation process.
2. Locations where the fertilization or experimentation is conducted.
3. Name and address of any persons, facility, agency sponsoring the fertilization or experimentation except that the names of any persons who are donors or recipients of sperm or eggs shall not be disclosed.
4. Number of eggs fertilized.
5. Number of eggs fertilized or destroyed or discarded.
6. Number of women implanted with a fertilized egg.

Any person required under this subsection to file a report, keep records or supply such information, who willfully fails to file such report, keep records or supply such information or who submits a false report shall be assessed a fine by the department in the amount of $50.00 for each day in which that person is in violation hereof.

have not yet been tested in the courts as applied to IVF. There currently are laws that ban or limit fetal and/or embryo research in twenty-five states (see table 5.2). Some of these laws conceivably could be applied to prohibit reproductive-mediating technologies, such as embryo donation, cryopreservation of embryos, or manipulation of the embryo. Twelve of these states have statutory provisions that can be interpreted to restrict sale or donation of em-

TABLE 5.2. Fetal Research—State Statutes

State	Restricts fetal research	Prohibits sale of fetus or embryo	Mentions preimplantation embryos(a)	May restrict research with pre-embryos(b)
Arizona	x		x	x
Arkansas	x	x		x
California	x		x	x
Florida	x	x		x
Illinois	x		x	x
Indiana	x			
Kentucky	x			x
Louisiana	x(c)		x	x
Maine	x		x	x
Massachusetts	x		x	x
Michigan	x		x	x
Minnesota	x		x	x
Missouri	x			
Montana	x			
Nebraska	x			
New Mexico	x		x	
North Dakota	x		x	x
Ohio	x	x	x	x
Oklahoma	x	x	x	x
Pennsylvania	x		x	x
Rhode Island	x		x	x
South Dakota	x			x
Tennessee	x	x		
Utah	x	x	x	x
Wyoming	x			x

Source: Adapted from OTA 1988a:251.

a. By terms such as "embryo," "product of conception," "conceptus," or "unborn child."
b. Statute could be interpreted as prohibiting some pre-embryo research.
c. Louisiana statute found unconstitutional in *Margaret S. v. Edwards* (1986).

bryos, whether created through in vitro or in vivo fertilization. Six of these states explicitly prohibit the sale of a fetus or embryo. Although it is yet unclear if all of these laws will be applied to IVF directly, five states currently specify this connection. The Illinois law, for instance, states that any person who unites the ovum and sperm outside the human body is deemed to have care and custody of the resulting child. The state supreme court (*Smith v. Hartigan,* 1983) subsequently interpreted this provision to mean that care and custody ended after transfer of the embryo to the woman, who then had care and custody.

The Legal Context of SM

In light of the Baby M. case in New Jersey, a number of state legislatures have introduced legislation specifically forbidding the practice of surrogate motherhood within their boundaries. A recent study found 73 bills on surrogacy in 27 states and the District of Columbia (Isaacs and Holt 1987:28). Twenty-five of the bills would have forbidden SM, 26 would regulate it, and 22 would create commissions to study it. A bill overwhelmingly passed by the Nevada assembly in 1989 would make SM legal, but establish a solid regulatory framework. It would require home visits of all parties by the state welfare division and proof that the intended mother was infertile. Both the surrogate mother and intended parents would be required to undergo counseling, testing for venereal disease, psychological exams, and genetic screening. In July 1987, Louisiana became the first state to enact a statute that makes SM contracts unenforceable. In June 1988, Michigan became the first state to make it a criminal offense to enter or arrange a surrogate contract and imposed substantial penalties of fines and imprisonment. In contrast, Arkansas passed legislation endorsing SM, Kansas exempts SM from prohibitions on adoption agency advertising, and Nevada specifically exempts SM from its prohibition on baby-selling.

Although the fate of most of these SM-specific bills is not yet determined, other more general statutes may affect this application. Thirty-six states currently prohibit payment beyond expenses in connection with adoption. Proponents of SM have argued that it is different from adoption, because the surrogate mother is being compensated for a service, not for the baby per se, so that it should not fall under baby selling laws. Critics of surrogate contracts contend it is no different and that such statutes should apply. Undoubtedly, court action in the individual states will do little to establish a consensus on this matter of interpretation. In the absence of clarified legislation that specifically exempts SM from these laws, however, parties to SM contracts are on very shaky legal ground at best.

Ironically, laws instituted to protect sperm donors from paternity, when applied to SM, complicate the legal status of the SM contract. In many states, the man who donates (or sells) the sperm to a woman who is not his wife is not the legal father of the child. If New Jersey had such a law, the claim of paternity for William Stern (which ultimately was the basis for his being awarded custody of Baby M.) would likely have been voided. This situation cogently demonstrates how complex and potentially confusing the legal context of reproductive technologies can become. By protecting the interests of one party under one application, that same party in a different application is deprived. The futility of writing legislation specific enough to be equitable yet general enough to make sense is obvious here.

State Legislation in Insurance Coverage for TMR

Although there currently are no comprehensive data on the proportion of TMR costs reimbursed by private insurers, an increasing number of carriers provide routine coverage for IVF and other TMR interventions if medically indicated (Toth, Washington, and Davis 1987). Many group plans that cover infertility services, however, do not pay for IVF on grounds that it is still experimental, although that rationale for exclusion is bound to weaken. This inconsistency in coverage of IVF from plan to plan has led to efforts by groups such as RESOLVE to lobby for state legislation that mandates third-party coverage.

As of 1987, five states (Arkansas, Hawaii, Maryland, Massachusetts, and Texas) had adopted legislation requiring insurance carriers to reimburse IVF and related services. In addition, at least five other states (California, Connecticut, Delaware, Washington, and Wisconsin) were considering such action during the 1988 legislative sessions.

Of the five states with statutes, Massachusetts has the most extensive. In 1987, it enacted legislation (Act H3721) requiring that all insurance plans that cover pregnancy-related benefits provide coverage for medically indicated expenses of diagnosis and treatment of infertility to the same extent that benefits are provided for other pregnancy-related procedures. Under the regulations promulgated under this act and in effect as of January 6, 1988, insurers must provide benefits for all nonexperimental infertility procedures. These include, but are not limited to, AI, IVF, and other procedures recognized as nonexperimental by the American Fertility Society (AFS), the American College of Obstetricians and Gynecologists (ACOG), or other infertility experts recognized by the state Commissioner of Insurance. Surrogacy, reversal of voluntary sterilization, and procurement of donor eggs and sperm are specifically excluded from coverage in the regulations. The insurers may establish reasonable eligibility requirements, which are to be made available to the insured.

The four remaining states all require coverage for IVF, but each state has some exemptions or limitations. Maryland, for instance, restricts coverage to persons who have been seeking infertility treatment for at least five years or with infertility associated with specific conditions. The use of IVF for couples with male-factor-only infertility is not covered. The person seeking IVF treatment must have exhausted all non-IVF treatments covered under the insurance plan. In addition to restrictions on eligibility similar to Maryland's, Hawaii requires coverage for one IVF cycle only, even though—practically speaking—four or five cycles are considered normal. In Texas, all plans that have maternity benefits must offer benefits for IVF, though the policy holder does not have to accept these benefits. Insurers affiliated with a bona fide religious denomination that objects to IVF for moral reasons are exempt from this requirement. Arkansas law sets a lifetime maximum benefit of $15,000, which may include other infertility benefits. Because a series of IVF alone may cost upwards of $20,000, beneficiaries are likely to have substantial personal investments.

Although the legislation in these states broadens accessibility to TMR, in no case is coverage extended to those persons least able to afford them, i.e., Medicaid recipients. The political ramifications of extending Medicaid coverage in these times of scarcity makes sense fiscally, but reinforces the inequity of access to TMR.

Most importantly, however, more than forty states have no policy concerning third-party coverage for TMR. As a result, there continues to be considerable inconsistency both within and across these states. For instance, employees under Blue Cross/Blue Shield in Delaware have an option to purchase IVF coverage (no minimum waiting period, $25,000 lifetime maximum). Furthermore, the Prudential medical insurance programs nationwide recognize infertility as an illness and routinely cover virtually all related services, including AIH and IVF, as long as the services conform to ACOG standards and are determined to be medically necessary (OTA 1988:151).

In the absence of state mandates, the majority of health insurance plans and HMOs exclude specific coverage for IVF. Its potentially high cost and its low success rate, combined with its perception as a procedure of uncertain benefit to the few at the expense of many, continues to deter many insurers from entering this market. It is not surprising, therefore, that those groups demanding such coverage have gone to the state legislatures for satisfaction. In those states where major efforts have been made, the success rate has been high.

Fertility Control Policy

In contrast to TMRs, sterilization has been at the center of the public policy process since the early 1900s. Unfortunately, the history of this policy area has been one of controversy, and legislation has usually focused on legalizing involuntary applications. In the United States, initial interest in sterilization was based on social control, not on the grounds of individual choice. Early legislation was motivated both by medical theories that postulated that mental illness was inherited and by elitist theories stemming from social Darwinism (Kevles 1986). In 1907, Indiana passed a Eugenic Sterilization Law that sought to eliminate retardation simply by sterilizing relevant target groups of "unfit" individuals. Eventually, thirty more states passed legislation that empowered mental and corrective institutions to sterilize inmates. In some states, such as Washington, statutes were extended to permit punitive sterilization of certain felons (especially those convicted of rape), chronic alcoholics, and derelicts.

The extent to which the eugenic logic dominated American society is reflected in Justice Oliver Wendell Holmes' affirmation in *Buck v. Bell* (1927) of the duty of the state to impose sterilization as

TABLE 5.3. State Legislation for Nonconsensual
Sterilization, 1988.

| | PERSONS ADDRESSED | |
State	Institutional Only	Private and Inst.
Arkansas		x
California		x
Colorado		x
Connecticut		x
Delaware		x
Idaho		x
Kentucky		x
Maine		x
Minnesota		x
Mississippi	x	
New Hampshire		x
North Carolina		x
North Dakota	x	
Oklahoma	x	
Oregon		x
South Carolina	x	
Utah		x
Vermont		x
Virginia		x
West Virginia		x

SOURCE: Association for Voluntary Surgical Contraception, 1988.

an appropriate exercise of its police power. Holmes' conclusion
that "three generations of imbeciles are enough" is a cogent re-
minder of how even faulty medical theory can influence the Court.
That decision's callous disregard for the rights of the individuals
concerned was not questioned until the Court in *Skinner v. Oklahoma* (1942) held that a state law authorizing involuntary sterilization of particular felons violated the right of equal protection.
According to Justice Douglas, marriage and procreation are civil
rights of man, fundamental to the very existence and survival of
the race:

The power to sterilize, if exercised, may have subtle, far-reaching
and devastating effects. . . .There is no redemption for the individual

INITIATOR			Court
	Parent or	Procedural	Order
Administrator	Guardian	Safeguards	Required
	x	x	x
	x	x	x
	x	x	x
x	x	x	x
x		x	
x	x	x	x
x		x	
x	x	x	x
x		x	
	x	x	x
x	x	x	x
x	x	x	x
x		x	
x	x	x	
x		x	
x		x	x
x	x	x	x
x	x	x	x
x	x	x	x

whom the law touches. Any experiment which the state conducts is to his irreparable injury. He is forever deprived of a basic liberty. Although *Skinner* did not address directly the question of eugenic sterilization, it raised procreative freedom to a fundamental right that cannot be readily violated.

Although the most glaring constitutional deficiencies have been recognized by the courts since *Skinner*, revised statutes (see table 5.3) permitting nonconsensual sterilization in limited cases have been upheld by a succession of courts. In California, a 1987 law authorizing sterilization for developmentally disabled persons was, in fact, motivated by the California Supreme Court when it declared unconstitutional a 1980 law banning sterilization of mentally retarded persons (*Conservatorship of Valerie N*). In most cases, the revisions in state legislation reflect a noticeable shift in rationale for sterilization from the largely discounted eugenic arguments to a concern for the best interests of the affected individuals or their potential progeny. Three related themes are apparent in the resurgence of proposed sterilization legislation since the 1970s. The first is the presumption that mentally retarded persons are incapable of being fit parents; therefore, to protect their potential as well as actual progeny, the retarded ought to be sterilized without their consent, since informed consent on their part is impossible. A second approach is paternalistic and argues that sterilization is in the best interest of the affected person. Menstrual periods and pregnancy represent unnecessary burdens on sexually active retarded women: by sterilizing them, society frees them from these emotional and physical burdens.

A third theme in some of the proposed legislation is directed toward women on public assistance and is utilitarian at its base. Welfare recipients unable themselves to control their fertility, it is argued, represent a drain on the taxpayers. To relieve what is perceived to be an unfair burden on the state in caring for numerous children when the parents have no responsibility or ability to do so, coerced sterilization has been proposed in at least ten states. Although none of the bills based on this latter argument has passed, persons on public assistance remain vulnerable. According to the Committee to Defend Reproductive Rights, poor women are sterilized at disproportionately higher rates than nonpoor women. For example, sterilization rates for women on welfare are 49 percent higher than those who are not. Moreover, people of color have been sterilized in substantially greater proportions than whites: 20 percent of black women, 24 percent of Native American women, 22 percent of Chicanos, 37 percent of Puerto Rican women, and 16 percent of white women were sterilized as of 1979. However, general public sentiment seems to favor such measures, and because many of the targets of such legislation are members of minority groups, the situation is politically sensitive.

Many reports of coerced operations have been made, and there are allegations that welfare workers have threatened recipients with a loss of benefits unless they agree to be sterilized. If the estimate of 200,000 federally funded sterilizations a year is accurate (Sewell 1980) it would be surprising if some of these were not coerced in some manner. Purportedly, women have been sterilized without their knowledge while they were in the hospital for abortions or other surgeries. After passage of the 1970 Family Planning Act made sterilization available in federally funded clinics, reports of many such abuses surfaced. And so, in response to the growing controversy, and in the absence of federal standards for voluntarism, the U.S. Department of Health, Education, and Welfare imposed in 1974 a moratorium on the federal funding of sterilization of all minors and those considered mentally incompetent. A subsequent district court injunction permanently enjoined the government from sterilizing minors and incompetents.

The department also went a step further and imposed guidelines on the sterilization of all other public assistance recipients. Individuals had to be informed of the nature, risks, and irreversible nature of sterilization. A waiting period of at least 72 hours was required between the written consent and the performance of the sterilization. Before consenting, the welfare recipient had to be informed that benefits could not be withdrawn if she or he refused to undergo the procedure. Furthermore, the sterilization had to be approved by a five-member review committee appointed by responsible authorities of the federally funded or sponsored (e.g., Medicaid) program or project.

The following federal requirements currently apply to all sterilizations funded in full or part by the U.S. government:

1. The candidate must be at least 21 years old, not be legally declared incompetent, give voluntary informed consent, and wait a minimum of 30 days but no longer than 80 days between signing the informed consent form and the sterilization.
2. The sterilization candidate must be given by the provider, orally or by videotape, information which includes available alternative methods of birth control, the risks and benefits of the procedure, the irreversibility and permanency of the procedure. Consent cannot be obtained during childbirth or labor, in relation to abortion, or under the influence of alcohol or drugs.
3. The informed consent form must be signed by the person seeking sterilization, the person who obtains the consent, the physician performing the sterilization, and an interpreter if relevant.

The availability of safe and effective sterilization techniques that promise high rates of reversibility and long-term subdermal implants such as NORPLANT will create a social climate in which pressures for voluntary, as well as nonconsensual, sterilization will heighten. Sterilization, then, no longer represents a permanent destruction of a person's reproductive capacity but, rather, a less intrusive and presumably temporary cessation of fertility. It is less difficult to rationalize the imposition of such temporary and less destructive procedures on any human, especially those for whom informed consent is not possible. From a purely technical standpoint, nonconsensual sterilization is more easily justified under such circumstances. However, these same innovations which promise to make sterilization less invasive technically also threaten to increase the frequency of its use for eugenic or social control purposes by eliminating its most offensive aspect—irreversibility.

The opponents of compulsory sterilization have long emphasized the irreversible nature of sterilization and given considerable weight to the "finality" of sterilization (*Skinner v. Oklahoma 1942*). Will the new reversible techniques also reverse the trend toward more stringent regulations on its use? Certainly, it is easier to justify a reversible procedure; but this capacity also raises such questions as who decides when to "pull the plug"? Is there much likelihood that the technically "reversible" sterilization will ever actually be reversed, or is the knowledge of that possibility enough? Should the government pay the costs of reversing sterilization, if it paid for or ordered the original procedure?

Sewell (1980:122) emphasizes that sterilization abuse "impacts on minority and poor women," and contends that the race and class nature of the abuse permeates the attitudes of health providers. Given the current negative attitudes of the public toward those on welfare, the increased emphasis on the population problem, the scarcity of public funds for welfare programs, and the emerging focus on the competency of parents, it would not be surprising if the availability of reversible sterilization gave impetus to pressures for widespread use of incentives (or coercion) to encourage (or force) sterilization of the poor, retarded, and those otherwise deemed "unfit."

Although attention has, most recently, returned to nonconsensual applications, during the 1960s and 1970s considerable debate has centered on the legal status of voluntary applications. At present, voluntary sterilization for adults capable of making an informed choice is legal in all 50 states. In order to regulate voluntary sterilization, however, some states have specific requirements that must be met prior to carrying out the procedure.

1. Age requirements for voluntary sterilization candidates include:
   A. In Arkansas, Maryland, Massachusetts, Nevada, North Carolina, Virginia, and West Virginia, voluntary sterilization of unemancipated minors is prohibited.
   B. In Rhode Island, sterilization of anyone under 18 is a felony except to preserve that person's life or health.
   C. In Georgia, married persons under 18 may obtain sterilization only under specific conditions.
   D. In New York City, the minimum age is 21.
2. A waiting period of 30 days between the time of informed consent and the sterilization is required in California, Virginia, and New York City.
3. Consent of spouse is required in Georgia, New Mexico, and Virginia.
4. Second-opinion consultation is required of physicians in Georgia and North Carolina.

In spite of these restrictions, most competent adults are now able to undergo contraceptive sterilization across the 50 states.

PRIVATE ASSOCIATION GUIDELINES FOR TMR

While state governments have slowly and cautiously entered the arena of TMR, private associations have issued guidelines to their members. The two most active organizations in promulgating relevant standards of practice are The American Fertility Society (AFS) and The American Association of Tissue Banks (AATB). The AFS is the fastest-growing subspecialty group in medicine, with membership of over 10,000. Since 1986, it has prepared a set of ethical guidelines to govern reproductive mediating-technologies, issued position papers on insurance coverage of infertility services, and published revised procedures for AID. Its journal, *Fertility and Sterility*, is a major source of information on TMR. Similarly, the AATB sets standards for tissue banking, including germ material. In 1986, it initiated a program of inspection and accreditation of tissue banks. It, along with AFS and the American College of Obstetricians and Gynecologists (ACOG), serves as quasi-public regulators of TMRs in the absence of government regulations.

Voluntary Guidelines for AID

In anticipation of further government intervention and an attempt
at self-regulation, two of these private organizations have issued
guidelines for AID practitioners. AFS and AATB are concerned with
assuring the credibility of AID services and maintaining quality
control among their member agencies. Most, although not all, professional services are affiliated with these associations. The most
recent AATB standards for tissue banking, approved in 1984, call
for the screening of donors for personality, for physical traits, and
for occupational factors associated with birth defects. Ideally, the
screening includes an "in-depth semen analysis which includes
microbial screening" and periodic testing for hepatitis and syphilis
(AATB 1984). They recommend that a man not be used as a sperm
donor if, according to his family history, he is at greater than 1
percent risk of producing a child with a genetic defect. The AFS
guidelines, published in 1986, recommend that AID be performed
only by a licensed physician; that donors be screened for genetic or
venereal disease, be under the age of 50, and sign consent forms
acknowledging use of their sperm for AID, and be assured that
their identity will be kept confidential. They also recommend that
physicians keep written records, that donors be absolved of any
rights or responsibilities to the child conceived through the use of
their sperm, that the child be considered legitimate, so that it may
enjoy the same rights as a naturally born child, and that the child
of AID is not the donor's child. Payment to donors will vary from
area to area, but it should not be such that the monetary incentive
is the primary factor in donating sperm. Because of the concern
over consanguinity that might result from widespread use of a
single donor's sperm, the guidelines set a limit at ten or less pregnancies per donor. (For a more detailed look at specific donor
screening criteria, see AFS 1986b:83S-86S.) In February 1988, AFS
issued revised guidelines in response to the AIDS epidemic. These
revisions (figure 5.2) call for exclusive use of frozen semen in all
AID services.

In addition to these formalized guidelines and the regulation in
a handful of states, individual sperm banks usually have their own
internal procedures that affect quality control. Some sperm banks
limit the number of children any one donor can sire in order to
prevent incestuous marriages between half-siblings. Most banks

now have procedures for genetic screening of potential donors and take medical histories for future use of the AID children.

Despite promising attempts at public as well as private initiatives in regulating AID services, a significant minority of them occur outside the professional context and are difficult to monitor. Moreover, there remain many questions concerning the liability of semen banks. For instance, what if they mislabel a deposit, resulting in the birth of a mulatto to two black parents (Reilly 1977:204)? What if the semen accidentally is destroyed by power failure or bankruptcy of the semen bank? What happens if a depositor fails to pay the annual storage fee? Since it appears that a greater proportion of semen banking in the future will take place in commercial enterprises, what guarantees does a depositor have as to continued service? These legal questions and many others are bound

---

FIGURE 5.2. Revised New Guidelines for the Use of
Semen-Donor Insemination

In response to increasing concerns regarding the possible transmission of the human immunodeficiency virus (HIV) during donor semen insemination and to the absence of a cure for this disease at present, The American Fertility Society is revising its New Guidelines for the Use of Semen-Donor Insemination: 1986. Since it is possible for the virus for acquired immune deficiency syndrome (AIDS) to be transmitted by fresh donor semen before the donor has become seropositive, a phenomenon which may take up to 3 months or possibly longer to occur after initial infection, the potential for transmission of human immunodeficiency virus (HIV) by fresh semen cannot be eliminated entirely. It is therefore The American Fertility Society's position that under present circumstances the use of fresh semen for donor insemination is no longer warranted and that all frozen specimens should be quarantined for 180 days and the donor retested and found to be seronegative for HIV before the specimen is released.

This position is consistent with our goal to provide maximum safety for our patients undergoing this procedure. We recognize that there may be some decrease in pregnancy rates and/or length of time to conceive when using frozen semen. We urge directed efforts be made to evaluate the true effectiveness of frozen semen and to improve cryopreservation techniques.

SOURCE: American Fertility Society 1988a:211.

to occur in the near future, again demonstrating the interaction of technology and society.

In the discussion of professional guidelines earlier, it was noted that the AATB guidelines for AID apply specifically to cryobank facilities. The standards emphasize that frozen semen is preferable to fresh because it allows adequate time for the requisite screening. In addition to the specifics on donor screening, the AATB recommends that all cryobanks be prepared to conduct a wide range of biochemical assays and chromosomal studies if requested by a physician. Furthermore, the AATB through its Reproductive Council proposed that it serve as the "instrument of requisite certification" of cryobanks. Although Frankel (1979:95) sees this as an important step in the direction of protecting recipients and progeny, many issues remain unresolved. Because the standards apply only to the use of frozen sperm by cryobanks, they do not affect fresh semen, which still accounts for the vast majority of AID. Nor does it cover the practices of physicians performing AID independent of banks. Moreover, although certification of semen cryobanks is valuable for those banks which join, as of now there is no reason for those operators not already committed to the aims of AATB to become members.

One means around this impasse is for states to require accreditation or certification of cryobanks. State licensing power could also be used on grounds of protecting the public health. Although such initiatives might emerge as cryobanks become more widespread, especially if critical legal questions are raised over their liability, there has been little interest in the state legislatures on this point. At this time, anyone with sufficient funds and proper equipment can open a cryobank. Commercialization trends in health care, particularly clinics, will increase competition and make attractive cost efficient shortcuts in the screening of donors and in record-keeping. Eventually, state action might be necessary in order to protect the integrity of existing sperm banks which until now has been fundamentally strong. One observer (Pendleton 1979) predicts that sperm bank advertisements soon might promote home-insemination kits, which less scrupulous cryobanks will sell directly to consumers. Thus, self-regulation by the emerging cryobank industry is unlikely to be effective in fully protecting women undergoing AID and their progeny.

As problems arise in the safety and, to a lesser extent, the efficacy of cryobanking practices of particular semen banks, the courts

undoubtedly will be asked to intervene. At that point, the existing
professional standards established by AATB and other associations
most likely will be used by the courts as guides to assessing legal
claims and liabilities. Banks that refuse to abide by the guidelines
will have to defend any of their actions at variance with them. In
the absence of accepted professional standards, the courts might
impose their own standards, as they do in other medical applications. This situation might compromise the availability of AID and
semen cryobanking and produce conflicting standards across legal
jurisdictions. Despite the current lack of applicability and enforce-
ment of cryobanking guidelines, they serve a valuable function and
a useful base upon which to build.

Voluntary Guidelines for IVF Centers

In 1986, an ad hoc committee of AFS issued minimal standards for
IVF programs (AFS 1986a:87S-88S). Every group initiating an IVF
program should have all aspects of the program approved by a
"properly constituted" institutional review board (IRB). The IRB
should ensure that a record is kept of all attempts made at securing
pregnancies by IVF including "all medical aspects of the treatment
cycles and a record of success or failure with respect to oocyte
recovery, fertilization, cleavage, conceptus transfer, biophysical
monitoring of fetal growth, pregnancy outcome, and complications" (AFS 1988a:87S). Furthermore, the guidelines recommend
that special attention be given to the emotional needs and support
of the patients.

The AFS guidelines recommend that the program director have
clinical experience and competence. At a minimum, the staff should
include persons trained with four types of skills: reproductive en-
docrinology; pelvic reparative surgery with laparoscopic experience; male reproduction; and experience in tissue culture, gamete
maturation, fertilization, and early zygote cleavage. Finally, an IVF
program should have the following services and facilities available
on a 24–hour, daily, basis: ultrasound, hormonal assays, facilities
for follicular aspiration and conceptus transfer, anesthesia, and
laboratory facilities with two-way communication to the operating
room. In 1984, the American College of Obstetricians and Gynecologists (1984) promulgated similar recommendations.

Along with its IVF program guidelines, AFS published an ethical statement to guide conduct in IVF clinics. A reading of the nine paragraphs in figure 5.3 shows that they largely address disposition of embryos including transfer, research, and cryopreservation. The AFS statement pronounces IVF, for infertility not solvable by other means, as ethically sound, calls for informed consent on the part of all parties, and approves of the use of donor sperm and ova for IVF. Again, as with all other guidelines of these associations, they are not legally binding even on the member programs. They are recommendations only, but in the absence of legislation they serve a valuable purpose. It is yet unclear as to whether voluntary compliance with association guidelines carries any protection against tort action, although it seems that noncompliance with what serve as professional standards might invite such action when harm occurs.

The AFS special interest group on IVF has recently formalized bylaws for the Society of Assisted Reproductive Technology (SART). Membership in this society requires a minimum of 40 treatment

---

FIGURE 5.3. American Fertility Society Ethical Statement on IVF

I. In vitro fertilization for infertility not solvable by other means is considered ethical.

II. It is understood that any couple entering into a program of in vitro fertilization will have discussed and signed a proper consent form covering the various steps in the procedure. It is understood that the gametes and concepti are the property of the donors. The donors therefore have the right to decide at their sole discretion the disposition of these items, provided such disposition is within medical and ethical guidelines as outlined herein.

III. In the event there are concepti in excess of those required for transfer in the harvest cycle, they may be treated at the option of the couple in accordance with paragraphs IV, V, or VII.

IV. It is considered ethically acceptable to scientifically examine any conceptus donated for this purpose, provided such examination is carried out prior to the time development has reached the stage when implantation would normally occur. For purposes of this paragraph, 14 days after insemination is considered to be the limit.

V. Nontransferred concepti should not be allowed to develop in the laboratory more than 14 days and may be disposed of without scientific examination.

cycles per year and at least three live births. SART members must comply with the AFS standards for personnel and facilities. In 1984, the AFS Committee on Ethics was charged with addressing ethical issues of the new reproductive technologies and providing disseminated knowledge of their positions. This distinguished committee of ethicists, lawyers, researchers, and clinicians issued its report in 1986 to serve as a framework for further discussion and deliberation (AFS 1986a). Finally, in 1988, AFS promulgated standards for gamete intrafallopian transfer (GIFT). According to AFS, GIFT may be considered a standard clinical procedure provided:

1. The patient and her partner have been investigated using as a minimum the standards established by the American Fertility Society.
2. The patient has at least one normal fallopian tube and a condition not amenable to less invasive techniques.

VI. Cryopreservation of concepti for the purpose of subsequent implantation into the female partner is acceptable with certain provisions. The concepti should not be retained in the cryopreserved state for longer than the reproductive life of the female donor. However, the disposition of any unused cryopreserved concepti should be provided for prior to cryopreservation and in accordance with the guidelines of paragraphs IV, V, or VII.

VII. After the reproductive problem has been resolved to the satisfaction of the donors, it is considered ethically acceptable to donate to another infertile couple nontransferred concepti, provided any claim to any resulting progeny is waived and provided strict anonymity between donors and recipients is assured as in any adoptive procedure.

VIII. Donor sperm should be looked upon as any other donor insemination technique and should be considered ethical and sound for those males that even with in vitro fertilization cannot fertilize normally.

IX. Donor oocytes should be considered ethical and sound for those females who have no oocytes or whose oocytes are not available by contemporary techniques.

3. The facility has a gamete laboratory and personnel that meets
   The American Fertility Society minimum standards for an in
   vitro fertilization program.

They conclude that it is preferable that GIFT be performed in a
facility that is prepared to carry out IVF as an alternative in the
event that during the procedure GIFT proved not to be feasible
(1988b:20).

Federal Initiatives toward Regulating TMRs

Congress is beginning to make long-overdue overtures in response
to the problem of regulating reproductive services. In 1987 and
1988, four separate House subcommittees held preliminary hearings on various aspects of TMRs. The Select Committee on Children, Youth, and Families (U.S. Congress 1987a) took testimony
from a wide range of experts on TMRs to explore the medical,
legal, and ethical issues with a particular focus on their implications for children and families. Also in 1987, the Subcommittee on
Civil Service (U.S. Congress 1987b) held hearings on the Federal
Employee Family-Building Act (HR 2852), which would address
inequities in access to TMRs by requiring all insurance carriers
offering obstetric coverage under the federal employee health benefits program to provide benefits for "family-building" procedures,
including IVF. With a similar focus, the Subcommittee on Human
Resources and Intergovernmental Relations of the House Committee on Government Operations began hearings on the federal role
in the prevention and treatment of infertility and the effects of the
roadblock on funding IVF research and infertility services.

The hearings on consumer protection issues involving IVF clinics, held by the Subcommittee on Regulation and Business Opportunities of the House Committee on Small Business (U.S. Congress
1988) hold the most promise of eventual action to address specifically the question of regulation. These hearings were motivated by
Chairman Wyden's (D. Ore.) concern with the lack of adequate
state regulation. Due to the de facto moratorium on federal funding
of IVF research, and the resulting lack of accountability and control that normally accompanies it, Congressman Wyden correctly
felt that some effort to institute federal oversight is necessary. The
hearings emphasized two areas of essential action: dissemination
of information to consumers and regulation.

In his testimony before the subcommittee, Richard Marrs, director of the Reproductive Center at Good Samaritan Hospital and a leading IVF practitioner and researcher, concluded that regulatory control is badly needed because of the proliferation of centers doing IVF. Professional guidelines, while useful, are voluntary and give no authority to dictate policy. As a result "there is no direct regulatory process" to protect the consumers and ensure quality care (U.S. Congress 1988:33). Marrs called for an established format for reporting pregnancy outcomes, an open registry to allow consumers to make educated decisions, standardization of laboratory facilities, and consistent licensing standards and regulations. The subcommittee surveyed all IVF centers in 1989 and published data in a booklet available to the public.

Similarly, interest in the regulation of AID services was sparked by an Office of Technology Assessment (1988a) report that showed that many practitioners were doing little to protect recipients from genetic disorders or infectious diseases. In introducing the report, Senator Albert Gore (D. Tenn.) stated that: "it is appalling that something as basic and essential as testing anonymous donors for the AIDS virus is not routinely done." He warned that if the Food and Drug Administration did not take appropriate steps to regulate screening and testing of donor semen, Congress would. Senator Gore was writing a bill to establish a national data bank to store the medical and genetic history of all donors. In addition to ensuring that children of AID have access to these data, the national registry could function to monitor the frequency of the use of each donor and regulate AID services.

Although these disparate congressional endeavors are laudable, they demonstrate once more the lack of a comprehensive, coordinated approach to making reproductive policy. The hearings clearly illustrate the tendency of each committee to focus on particular aspects of the problem to the exclusion of many others. Also, by concentrating on one or several applications, the cumulative impact of reproductive and genetic technologies is obscured. Even if these hearings result in federal legislation or motivate regulatory responses from the states, they fail to deal with the harder questions concerning social priorities in reproduction and the directions we, as a society, want to take. Despite this, the new attention of Congress to reproductive issues is encouraging and reflects a recognition of their growing policy importance.

CONCLUSIONS: CURRENT REGULATIONS
AND STANDARDS

Although the standards promulgated by professional organizations are valuable and provide some control over the use of TMRs, the problem with guidelines as opposed to regulation is that there is no authority behind the guidelines to ensure compliance. Instead of the force of law, association guidelines rely on creditation privileges and ethical sanctions. There is, however, little to stop the establishment of nonaccredited or nonsanctioned cryobanks, fertility clinics, or IVF/GIFT/SM services. Although lack of compliance with the guidelines by nonmember businesses carries some risk, in the emerging highly lucrative commercial fertility industry, voluntary guidelines might not be a strong enough form of self-enforcement or policing of such activities. At the least, what is needed is some force of law to ensure that these standards apply to all TMR services.

The inadequacy of current state legislation to regulate effectively reproductive technologies (other than sterilization perhaps) is obvious. Even as clear and uncontroversial an issue as screening donor sperm to assure the health of the AID child has largely been ignored by all but several states. Thus far, the states have failed to provide any legal controls on the delivery of TMR services, even though they have the authority through licensing to do so. More importantly, in all but a handful of states, there appears to be little inclination for proactive policy making in this area. Recent interest in AIDS and IVF by several congressional committees demonstrates an awareness of these regulatory gaps and the possibility of a federal response to fill them.

In order to deal with the problems raised in chapters 3 and 4, coordinated governmental involvement is necessary. It appears unlikely that such action will be forthcoming from the individual states without encouragement from the federal government. The remainder of this book focuses on the development of a national policy to establish uniform minimal standards for research, application, and marketing of reproductive technologies. In this regard, the lessons learned from the experiences of other countries in dealing with these issues are critical. Therefore, before turning to U.S. national policy, the discussion in chapter 6 is devoted to the current status of international policy.

CHAPTER SIX

Comparative National Programs: What Can We Learn?

*T*HE POLITICAL culture of the U.S., with its heavy emphasis on rights, ensures that any attempts to regulate reproduction technologies will be designed specifically for that context. One cannot, for this reason, apply policy initiatives of other countries directly to the U.S., although the basic issues surrounding these technologies are similar across cultures. It is nevertheless valuable to analyze the experiences of other countries' efforts to establish reproduction policy. Until now, few attempts have been made to scrutinize the similarities, differences, and implications of action taken by other countries, many of which have moved much faster in this direction. This chapter analyzes and synthesizes those aspects of existing laws, commission reports, and issues papers that might be valuable for framing a draft policy for the United States.

REPRODUCTIVE TECHNOLOGY: AN EMERGING
INTERNATIONAL POLICY AREA

Given the political implications of the reproductive revolution, it
is not surprising that TMRs have engendered considerable public
debate in more than forty countries. Although public action in
most of these countries has been limited and actual public policy
initiatives rare, activities directed toward developing a national
response to these technologies in several countries are far more
advanced than in the United States.

Those countries with the most ambitious policy initiatives regarding TMRs are western nations that have a parliamentary system, in which the government in power is largely able to set the
agenda. Australia, Britain, and Canada seem to have taken the
lead, although several other countries, including Germany, France,
Israel, New Zealand, South Africa, and Sweden, have had major
national efforts to frame policy on these issues. After a review of
these actions, the cumulative implications for a national policy
and international guidelines will be analyzed.

General Approaches

The public mechanisms used to cope with the ethical, legal, and
political issues raised by reproductive technologies vary widely
across these countries and states. Appendix A lists some of the
major international efforts although—because of the rapid developments in this area—it is bound to be dated. Primarily, these
activities represent a combination of legislation, administrative
regulations, reports of commissions or other ad hoc bodies, and
court opinions. Legislation, both federal and state, has been adopted
in some countries to deal with particular techniques or applications. In some cases, the appropriate legislation is new, while in
other cases existing legislation such as family law, adoption law,
and criminal codes has been adapted, extended, or interpreted to
apply. In parliamentary systems, government White Papers or Consultation Papers, which often serve as the basis for future bills,
continue to serve as guidelines until legislation is passed. Other
bases of control are public health and licensing regulations, issues
papers, and departmental reports.

In most jurisdictions, the initiative for regulations and legislation has come from the reports of various forms of national commissions, legislative standing committees, and departmental committees (e.g., the Warnock Commission in Britain and the Waller Committee in Australia). In some cases, extensive hearings and public dialogue has accompanied the actions of these bodies. In other countries, the initiative has come from national medical associations, medical societies, or independent health councils. Some of these attempts at self-regulation have resulted in placing the issues on the public agenda. Alternately, in several cases these professional guidelines have become de facto public policy. Finally, in the absence of enabling legislation or regulations, the courts in a few countries continue to be the most visible source of policy making in response to reproductive technologies.

Warnock Committee

The progression of activity from committee to regulation is nowhere better exemplified than by developments in Great Britain since 1982. Undoubtedly, the single most influential report and one that sets the agenda for action in other countries began with the Warnock Committee. It is no surprise that Great Britain, the birthplace of the first IVF baby in 1978, produced the first comprehensive government-sponsored report on TMRs and reproductive research. In July 1982, the Warnock Committee was established by Parliament to consider evidence and make recommendations on issues in human assisted reproduction. Under the direction of its chairman Dame Mary Warnock, on June 25, 1984, the Committee made 64 separate recommendations for dealing with these emerging ethical and legal issues.

Overall, the tone of the Warnock Committee report is optimistic and sympathetic to the needs of infertile couples. It also recognizes the importance of regulatory oversight of these technologies and an active government role in the treatment of infertility.

As we have said, it would be idle to pretend that there is not a wide diversity in moral feelings, whether these arise from religious, philosophical or humanist beliefs. What is common (and this too we have discovered from the evidence) is that people generally want *some principles or other* to govern the development and use of the new techniques. There must be *some* barriers that are not to be crossed, *some* limits fixed, beyond which people must not be allowed to go. (Warnock Commission 1984:2)

To that end, the Committee recommended creation of a new statutory licensing authority (SLA) to regulate both research and infertility services:

1. A new statutory licensing authority be established to regulate both research and those infertility services which we have recommended should be subject to control.
2. There should be substantial lay representation on the statutory authority to regulate research and infertility services and that the chairman must be a layperson.
3. All practitioners offering the services we have recommended should only be provided under license, and all premises used as part of any such provision, including the provision of fresh semen and banks for the storage of frozen human eggs, semen and embryos should be licensed by the licensing body.

Specifically, the Warnock Committee recommended that AID, IVF, egg donation, embryo donation, the clinical use of frozen embryos, research on human embryos (up to 14 days after fertilization), and possible trans-species fertilization be permitted under licensing. Conversely, embryo donation by lavage should not be used at the present time and the use of frozen eggs in therapeutic procedures should not be undertaken until research has shown that no unacceptable risk is involved. The licensing authority shall review the data as it evolves. Furthermore, the sale or purchase of human gametes or embryos should be permitted only under license from and subject to conditions prescribed by the SLA.

In addition to the recommendations regarding licensing and control, the committee enumerated principles of provision designed to protect the public interest. First, sufficient public funding should be made available for the collection of adequate statistics on infertility and infertility services. Second, each health authority should review its facilities for the investigation and treatment of infertility and consider the establishment of a specialist infertility clinic with close working relationships with specialist units, including genetic counseling services, at regional and supraregional levels. Third, the committee recommended establishment of a working group at national level made up of central health departments, health authorities, and persons working in infertility, to draw up detailed guidance on the organization of services. The committee also urged that consideration be given to the inclusion of plans for infertility services as part of the next round of health authority strategic plans.

These principles of provision call for anonymity of donors, availability of counseling to all couples and third parties, accessibility of the child upon reaching age 18 to information about the donor's ethnic origin and genetic health, and informed consent of all parties. More specifically, there should be a limit of ten children who can be fathered by one donor, a gradual move towards a system where semen donors are given expenses only, and continued use of frozen semen in AID. All semen and egg deposits should undergo automatic five-year reviews, with a set maximum of ten years for the storage of embryos, after which time, the right to use or disposal should pass to the storage facility. As noted earlier, the Warnock Committee is unmatched in the comprehensiveness of its recommendations. Recommendation 29 even anticipates the marketing of "do-it-yourself" sex selection kits and places them under the "ambit of control" provided by the Medicines Act, with the aim of ensuring that such products are safe, efficacious, and of an acceptable standard for use.

The Warnock Committee would allow research on the human embryo and new infertility treatments, but only within legally established limits (recommendations 42 to 50). Most importantly, the committee sees violation of these legal strictures as constituting a criminal offense, presumably carrying severe sanctions. Because such services would fall under the National Health Service and the new licensing body, control would be more centralized than in the United States.

Finally, the committee recommended 14 legal changes. Many of these deal with clarifying the legitimacy of children born through AID and IVF. Several other recommendations involve specifics of succession and inheritance when these techniques are used. Recommendation 62 calls for the enactment of legislation to "ensure there is no right of ownership in a human embryo." The recommendations of the committee for legislation prohibiting surrogacy agreements (on which there was an expression of dissent in cases of last resort, Warnock Committee 1984:87) is the strongest call for the prohibition of any application in this document. As is evident from recommendations 57 to 59, the committee determined that surrogate contracts were contrary to the public good.

57. Legislation should be introduced to render criminal the creation or the operation in the United Kingdom of agencies whose purposes include the recruitment of women for surrogate pregnancy or making arrangements for individuals or couples who wish to utilise the services of a carrying mother; such legislation should be wide enough to include both profit and nonprofit making organisations.
58. Legislation should be sufficiently wide enough to render criminally liable the actions of professionals and others who knowingly assist in the establishment of a surrogate pregnancy.
59. It be provided by statute that all surrogacy agreements are illegal contracts and therefore unenforceable in the courts.

Overall, then, the Warnock Committee laid the groundwork for significant legislative activity in response to the new technologies of reproduction. The first response of the British Parliament to the Warnock Committee Report was to ban commercial surrogacy. The rapidity of this specific action, however, was spurred by one highly publicized court case involving a product of commercial surrogacy, the Baby Cotton case (Brahams 1987). Other issues raised by the Warnock Report, lacking such a dramatic case, were seen as requiring substantially more public dialogue. The call for further consultation on these issues was initiated by a Consultation Paper issued by the Department of Health and Social Security (1986). In November 1987, in response to public input up to June of that year, the government issued a White Paper that will serve as the basis for future legislation.

In concurrence with the Warnock Report, the White Paper of 1987 proposed a Statutory Licensing Authority (SLA) to oversee:

1. any treatment or research involving human embryos created in vitro or taken from the womb of the woman (e.g., lavage)
2. treatments involving donated gametes or embryos
3. the storage by cryopreservation of human gametes or embryos for later use
4. the use of diagnostic tests involving fertilization of an animal ovum by human sperm

The SLA is also to be responsible for licensing and collecting data on facilities offering reproductive techniques. It will maintain a central record of all gamete and embryo donations and births resulting from these donations. It will set and regulate the number of donations from any one donor and be responsible for ensuring that any financial transactions are limited to the recovery of reasonable costs only. The White Paper states that use of any of these techniques without the appropriate license is a criminal offense.

The British experience, although by far the most extensive at the federal level, is no longer unique in western democracies. The revolutionary nature of these new interventions has triggered considerable governmental activity across a wide array of related issue areas. Instead of proceeding on a country-by-country summary of action, at this point it is more useful to discuss cumulative activity for the specific techniques. The four areas that have thus far engendered the most policy activity are AID, IVF, SM, and human embryo research. Each is examined, in turn, below.

ARTIFICIAL INSEMINATION BY DONOR

At least 35 countries have either legislation, regulations, or guidelines concerning the practice of AID. Table 6.1 illustrates the major issues surrounding AID which have been addressed by governmental action and shows what mode of control is presently in use in each country. About half of these countries have legislation or regulations regarding AID, while the remainder depend primarily on commission reports or professional guidelines.

Is AID Allowed?

The first policy decision, and one which shapes the need for further action, is whether the practice of AID is allowed. As demonstrated in table 6.1, only three of these countries prohibit the practice of AID under all circumstances. The 1957 Code of Medical Rules in Brazil bans AID, although it permits AIH if both spouses consent to the procedure. In Egypt, too, AIH is allowed but AID is not. The most extreme negative response to AID is that of Libya where it is a criminal offense. The person who arranges or inseminates a woman, the woman herself, and her husband if he consents to the procedure, are all subject to imprisonment under Libya's criminal code. Unlike Brazil and Egypt, it is unclear whether AIH is permitted under Libyan law.

TABLE 6.1. Artificial Insemination

Country	Mode of Control of AID	AID Child Legitimate	Couples Only	Licensed Facilities Only
Australia	states	yes	couples	
Austria	report	yes	couples	
Belgium	legislation	yes		
Brazil	prohibit AID			
Bulgaria	legislation	yes	couples	
Canada	committee	yes	couples	yes
Chile	prof. guide			
Czechoslovakia	legislation	yes	couples	
Denmark	commission			yes
Egypt	prohibit AID			
FRG	reports	unc.	married	
Finland	practice			
France	commission	yes	couples	
GDR	practice	yes		yes
Greece	legislation	yes		
Hungary	legislation	yes		
Iceland	commission			
India	practice			
Ireland	prof. guide		married	
Israel	regulations	yes	married	yes
Italy	regulations		married	yes
Japan	prof. guide	yes		
Libya	prohibit AID			
Mexico	practice			
Netherlands	council	yes		
New Zealand	legislation	yes		
Norway	legislation	yes	couples	yes
Poland	courts	yes		
Portugal	regulations			yes
South Africa	regulations		married	yes
Spain	commission	yes	singles	yes
Sweden	legislation	yes	couples	yes
Switzerland	commission	yes		yes
United Kingdom	legislation	yes	couples	
Yugoslavia	legislation	vary		

Screening Donors-STDs	Screening Donors-Genetic	Records Required	Payment to Donor	Limit on Number Per Donor	Donor Secret
yes	yes	yes	varies	yes	
		yes		10	yes
			no		yes
	yes				yes
yes	yes	yes	expenses		yes
	yes				yes
					yes
		yes	no	1–10	
yes	yes		no		yes
			no		
yes	yes				yes
yes	yes	yes		yes	yes
yes					
		yes	yes		yes
yes	yes		no	yes	yes
yes					
					yes
			no		yes
yes	yes	yes		5	
yes	yes	yes		6	yes
		yes			child
	yes	yes			yes
		yes	expenses	yes	yes
			no		yes

Legitimacy of AID Children

In those countries which allow the practice of AID, a major concern centers on the legal status of the children born through AID. This, of course, is a critical issue because, without clarification of the child's status, the status of the donor is also questionable. Although the wording varies, most of the countries that have adopted laws on AID specify that, if the husband consents to the procedure, the resulting child is considered his legitimate offspring. A 1987 Belgian law, for instance, states that the child of AID with consent of the husband is legitimate and that the consenting husband cannot challenge paternity. Likewise, a 1983 Greek law states that the husband who has consented to his wife's undergoing AID cannot disavow paternity of the resulting child. The Family Law of Czechoslovakia states that the consenting husband may not contest paternity if the child is born six to ten months after AID. Similarly, the 1985 Swedish AI Law requires written consent of the husband or cohabitant of a woman undergoing AID, who as a result is regarded as the legal father. Bulgaria's Family Code also states that the consenting husband cannot later contest paternity.

In those countries without legislation, most committees and courts have recommended that laws be enacted to legitimize the children of AID. A report of a Canadian Advisory Committee on Storage and Utilization of Human Sperm urged that the child be considered the legitimate offspring of the woman and her consenting husband. Provincial reports reinforced this recommendation. Similarly, directives of the Council of Medical Research in Norway (1983) state that AID children should be considered legitimate. In Austria, a recent study recommended that AID be used only if the husband or partner is sterile and all parties give informed consent. If so, paternity cannot be contested after the fact. In Poland, a Supreme Court decision (1984) denied the consenting husband's challenge of paternity following AID. In Germany, in the absence of legislation, two conflicting court decisions have left the status of AID children unclear, although the later decision gave the consenting husband no right to contest the legitimacy and paternity of the resulting child.

There is developing consensus among those countries which allow AID that written consent of the husband or partner of the woman undergoing AID is essential if the child's legal status is to be assured. In many countries, however, this does not guarantee that a lawsuit over custody will never be filed, but consent makes it unlikely such a suit will be successful. In South Africa, permission of the donor's wife is also required and, in France, the sperm donor must be married and of proven fertility.

Access to AID Services

The emphasis placed on consent raises another issue—who should have access to AID services? As demonstrated in table 6.1, almost all countries that have addressed this issue limit AID either to married couples or unmarried couples in a stable relationship. Sometimes, as in the case of France—which limits AID to stable couples, but only if the male is sterile or has a genetic disorder—other restrictions are present. The Santosuosso Report (1984) in Italy proposed that donor insemination be limited to married couples and available only when adoption is not granted within six months of application. In Sweden, AID should be made available only if the prospective parents are of a character that enables the child to grow up under favorable conditions.

The question of allowing single or lesbian women access to AID has been approached explicitly in few jurisdictions and rejected in virtually all. A special commission in Spain recommended that single women be able to receive donor sperm for insemination if they can demonstrate the capability to provide an adequate home. Ontario's Law Reform Commission report on artificial reproduction (1985) would restrict access to "stable single women and to stable men and stable women in stable marital or nonmarital unions." A proposed law in Spain would permit the use of artificial reproduction techniques by homosexuals. No bill or government report from any other country was found to indicate government sympathy for use by lesbians, despite a demand (1986) by the Feminist International Network of Resistance to Reproductive and Genetic Engineering (FINRRAGE) that calls for "repudiation of legislative measures which would block access by certain groups of the population (for example single or lesbian women) to measures such as artificial insemination by donors."

Access to AID can also be circumscribed by legal constraints as to where it may be performed. Such restrictions, which are found in approximately ten countries, also enable administrators to monitor and regulate the practice more easily. The two general approaches are to require that AID services be performed either in public facilities or by licensed practitioners. In Norway, for instance, a 1987 law demands that AID be performed only at designated hospitals, with special authorization from the Ministry of Social Affairs and under the direction of trained specialists. Similarly, a 1985 Swedish law mandates that AID be performed in general hospitals and under the supervision of obstetrician/gynecologists.

AID in the German Democratic Republic is practiced in special infertility centers only, while, in Portugal, AID is available in publicly created centers or by private doctors who have been specially licensed by the Ministry of Health. Likewise, under Ministry of Health regulations in Israel, AID may be carried out only by a licensed obstetrician or gynecologist after thorough examination of both the husband and wife. Finally, South African regulations limit the practice of AID to physicians who are registered and approved by the Director General of the Department of National Health and Population Development. In addition, the physician is required to maintain detailed records of each donor and recipient, transfer of gametes, and health of the children born by AID. These records form the data base for an annual report to the Director General who maintains a central registry.

Regulations Over AID Services

In addition to potential state control over what agencies or persons can perform it, public health regulations can be initiated to specify how they perform it. About one-third of the countries that have addressed the issue of AID (see table 6.1) require screening of donors—for sexually transmitted diseases (10), for genetic disorders (11), or both (8). Also, because of the threat of the transmission of AIDS through AID, other countries are taking steps toward screening. In South Africa, recipients are screened for the same conditions as the donor to ensure they are suited for AID "biologically, physically, socially, and mentally." They must also be advised by the physician of the psychological and legal risks of AID.

Although payment for sperm donors is routine in the United States, most countries that have addressed the issue reject payment. Only Japan allows payment beyond expenses. The Ontario

Commission report recommends that donors be paid reasonable expenses as do the state committee reports in Australia. The Health Council of the Netherlands allows travel expenses only. In contrast, Belgium, France, Portugal, and Yugoslavia do not permit any compensation, while the German Democratic Republic has outlawed the sale or purchase of human gametes. Moreover, in some countries, such as New Zealand, the issue of payment for human sperm or ova has not arisen because of a strong tradition of voluntarism.

Another area of concern in regulation of AID services centers on the question of whether there should be limits on the number of times the semen of a particular donor can be used in order to reduce the chances of consanguinity. To date, at least eight countries have accepted the principle of setting limits although only several have actually specified the number of children allowed (South Africa, 5; Spain, 6; Austria, 10; and West Germany, 1 or 10, depending on which report recommendations are accepted). Because of its small population and, thus, heightened concern over this issue, Iceland imports all its sperm from Denmark.

Records and Access to Them

Most of the countries which have dealt in-depth with AID (through legislation, regulation, or comprehensive reports) require detailed record-keeping, although they differ as to what should be done with the information. Although most of the countries that require extensive records about the donor state that complete anonymity is essential, the Benda report in Germany concludes that the child conceived through AID should have access to this record when he or she turns 16 years of age. The 1985 AI law in Sweden requires that information about the sperm donor be kept on special hospital record for at least 70 years. At the age of 18, the child has a right to learn the identity of its biological father. In effect, the law equates AID with adoption, giving the donor a socially recognized position, but with no rights. Furthermore, the public welfare committee is duty bound to assist the child in retrieving this information. Although the parents are not obliged to disclose to the child the use of AID in his or her conception, the National Board of Health and Welfare encourages them to do so. According to Tranoy (1988:9), this action has brought the practice of AID to a virtual standstill in Sweden.

Few other countries appear inclined to take steps in the direction of Sweden. In Austria, records about the donor are confidential, although nonidentifying medical facts are revealed to the recipients or resulting children if necessary. Under Israeli regulations, strict records of the sperm donor are kept, but the identity of the donor remains confidential. As noted above, the SLA in Britain is to maintain a central record of all donor inseminations. At age 18, the child has access to nonidentifying information only. A similar system of record keeping has been recommended by the select commission in Spain, as well as by most state committees in Australia and Canada. Attesting to the detail of record-keeping under South Africa's regulations, recipients have access to nonidentifying information including the donor's age, height, weight, eye/hair color, complexion, population group, nationality, religion, occupation, education, and interests.

As regulations in these and other countries mature, a movement toward central registries is likely. This will serve as a means of monitoring the number of times a donor is used, as well as ensuring adequate record-keeping of the growing number of AID facilities. In those countries where the practice of AID is tightly controlled and channeled through public institutions, the task will be simpler. In those countries more similar to the U.S. where most AID is conducted outside the public sphere, the task will be considerably more difficult.

IN VITRO FERTILIZATION

Although IVF is a much more recent phenomenon than AID and presents considerably more complex policy issues, activity regarding IVF in many countries mirrors that of AID. To a large extent, the rapid developments in IVF and its extensions into embryo research motivated governmental response to the whole range of reproductive issues including AID. While some committees attempted to deal with the package of "artificial reproduction" technologies, increasingly more attention has been focused on the far-reaching implications of the ability to move conception from the womb to the laboratory.

Despite the more extensive ramifications of IVF than AID, the initial concerns are similar. They include questions surrounding the acceptability of the technique itself, the use of donor gametes and embryos, restrictions on recipients, regulation and licensing of facilities, record-keeping, and counseling. Additional issues center on the use of frozen embryos and their storage.

As illustrated in table 6.2, IVF utilizing the gametes of the recipient couple enjoys consensual support across these countries. Even in Greece, where IVF is illegal, it is practiced as a medical procedure. And in Egypt, where AID is forbidden, IVF using a married couple's own gametes is acceptable. Most countries that approve IVF specify approval only as treatment for infertility. In Austria and Italy, for example, committees recommend support for IVF only as treatment for infertility, and then only after other therapeutic techniques have proven unsuccessful. In Spain, the special committee stated that IVF should be available only to overcome infertility or to avoid a grave hereditary disorder. Other uses should be legal but not paid for by public funds. Likewise, in Norway, IVF is to be used only if the woman is otherwise sterile. At the state level, the Ontario Law Reform Commission and all Australian state committees found IVF acceptable but only for medical reasons.

There is some drop in support for IVF when donor gametes or embryos are used. In Norway, a 1987 law states that the couple's own gametes must be used and the intended rearing mother must carry the child. The Swiss Academy of Medical Sciences' directives state that IVF with donor gametes is not allowed. Moreover, transfer of embryos from one woman to another is prohibited. In Germany, the Benda report recommends IVF use only by married couples using their own gametes, but it opens the possibility for exceptions. For instance, surplus embryos after IVF might be implanted in another woman with the explicit consent of the donor couple. Not surprisingly, in Ireland, the Medical Council (1985) authorized IVF for married couples only, and only if all embryos are placed in the genetic mother during that single procedure (no freezing of embryos for future use is allowed). Recommendations in Italy allow donor sperm and ova, but not donor embryos, for use by married couples who are well informed about the risks.

Some jurisdictions, however, have accepted use of donor gametes and embryos. The Federal Law Council in Australia finds donor gametes acceptable but urges stronger standards and guidelines. They did not approve of the use of known related embryo donors, however. Children born from donor gametes should have access to nonidentifying information about their genetic parents before age 18 and identifying information after age 18. All of the

TABLE 6.2. Government Action and
New Reproductive Technologies

	IN VITRO FERTILIZATION						
	Couples gametes	*Donor gametes*	*Regulation, guidelines, licensing*	*Restriction on recipients*	*Records required*	*Counseling required*	*Use of frozen embryos*	*Limits on storage of frozen embryos*
Australia (Federal)	yes	yes	yes	couple	yes	yes	yes	y-unspec
New South Wales	yes	yes	yes	couple	yes	yes	yes	
Queensland	yes	yes	yes	couple	yes	yes	yes	
S. Australia	yes	no	yes	couple	yes	yes	yes	y-unspec
Tasmania	yes	yes	yes	couple	yes	yes	yes	
Victoria	yes	yes	yes	married	yes	yes	yes	y-unspec
W. Australia	yes	yes	yes	couple	yes	yes	yes	
Austria	yes	yes		couple			yes	3 years
Canada (National)								
Ontario	yes	yes	yes	couple			yes	10 years
Chile	yes			couple				
Denmark								
Egypt	yes			couple				
FRG	yes	no	yes	couple			limited	2 years
France	yes		prop				yes	1 year
German Demo. Rep.	yes	yes					limited	
Greece	no							
Ireland	yes	no		married			no	
Israel	yes	sperm	yes	cou/sin	yes	yes	yes	5–10 yrs
Italy	yes	yes	yes	married				
Japan	yes	no		married				
Mexico	yes	no		couple			yes	
Netherlands	yes		yes	couple			yes	
New Zealand	yes	no	yes	couple				
Norway	yes	no	yes	couple	yes		yes	1 year
South Africa	yes	yes	yes	couple	yes	yes	yes	
Spain	yes	yes	yes	couple			yes	5 years
Sweden	yes	no		couple				
Switzerland	yes	no	yes					
United Kingdom	yes	yes	yes	couple	yes	yes	yes	5 years

Australian state committees, except South Australia, accept the use of donor embryos. In Austria, a government study has recommended that couples should have access to IVF using donated eggs or embryos but only after all other treatment possibilities are exhausted, the husband consents, the egg has been fertilized with the

| | HUMAN EMBRYO RESEARCH | | | |
Commercial surrogate motherhood	*Use of spare embryos*	*Production of embryos for research*	*Time limits after fertilization*	*Review by board or committee*
no	no	no		
no	no	no		
no	no	no		
no	no	no		
no	no	no		
no	yes	no	14 days	
no	yes	no	14 days	
no	yes		14 days	yes
	yes	no	14–17 d	yes
yes	yes	yes	14 days	
no				
no	no	no		
no				
no	no	no		
no	yes	no	7 days	
no				
no				
no	no	no		
no	yes	no		
no	no	no		
no	yes		14 days	
no	yes			yes
no				
no				
no	yes		14 days	yes
no	yes	no	14 days	yes
no	yes	yes	14 days	yes
no	no	no		
no	yes	no	14 days	yes

husband's sperm, and if the woman is less than 45 years of age. Furthermore, cryopreservation of spare embryos is acceptable for future use by the couple, for embryo donation, or for research with permission of the parents.

As is evident from this discussion, most countries approving IVF restrict its use to stable couples—in several cases, married couples. The only exception is Israel, where 1987 Ministry of Health regulations allow eligibility of a single woman for IVF, but only if a social worker certifies that she is psychologically and economically able to raise a child. For this reason, Israel allows the use of donated sperm, though donation of ova to single women is not permitted. Although cryopreservation of embryos is allowed (up to ten years with special consent) in Israel, they must be transferred only to the genetic mother.

Table 6.2 shows that only Ireland explicitly rejects the use of frozen embryos in IVF. The Ontario Commission approves gamete banks but only if they operate under federal license and limit storage to ten years. Payment from users to defray reasonable costs and provide a reasonable profit is acceptable to the Commission. The National Health and Medical Research Council (NHMRC) in Australia also approves of embryo cryopreservation but only if limits are set on their storage. Recommendations in Austria would prohibit implantation of embryos after they have been frozen for three years, while a 1987 law in Norway sets the limit at one year.

The 1986 national committee in France considered embryo freezing an experimental procedure to be performed only under strict conditions in licensed centers with a one-year limit on storage. Similarly, the West German Benda Report states that freezing of human embryos can be considered only when embryo transfer is not immediately possible. Cryopreservation storage is limited to two years maximum, though the preference is for transfer during the woman's following cycles in order to improve the embryo's prospect of implantation.

Reports or regulations in four countries (including all six Australian states) require counseling of the couple. Five jurisdictions stipulate that adequate records of each application be kept. In Canada, the federal government maintains a central registry to keep track of IVF children. In South Africa, regulations state that IVF be performed only at licensed facilities, the number of which are to be restricted. In Sweden, IVF services are limited to general hospitals unless special permission from the National Board of Health and Welfare is secured. The Ontario Commission states that IVF be provided as an insured service but only at designated centers.

The most formalized guidelines for IVF centers were authorized by the Australian NHMRC. Under these guidelines, every institution offering IVF must have the program approved by an institutional ethics committee that includes at least five persons (lay-woman, layman, minister, lawyer, and medical graduate with research experience). One responsibility of the committee is to ensure that proper records are maintained. These and other guide-lines being developed in France, Israel, Canada, as well as Great Britain, should be read carefully by decision makers in the U.S. before they establish a regulatory framework for the practice of IVF.

The volatility of IVF policy is clearly illustrated by recent devel-opments in Australia, which maintained a dominant position in infertility research during the 1980s. In 1989, separate actions by the Victoria state government and the federal government threat-ened to retard IVF dramatically. First, in order to close a loophole in a state law prohibiting experimentation on human embryos older than 22 hours that allowed the testing of two-day-old IVF embryos prior to transfer, the state health minister declared a temporary moratorium on all embryo experimentation until the law could be thoroughly reviewed. Meanwhile, funding for IVF research was slashed and federal subsidies for IVF treatment, which until then covered about 30 to 50 percent of the cost of each IVF cycle in Australia, were reduced in part because of questions con-cerning its cost effectiveness in treating infertility (Scott 1989:4).

COMMERCIAL SURROGACY

Unlike other applications of reproductive technology, surrogate motherhood enjoys no support in other nations, thus largely limit-ing its practice to the United States. This is especially so for com-mercial surrogacy enterprises or any other exchange of money. Table 6.2 demonstrates that all jurisdictions except Ontario reject commercial surrogacy. Moreover, most disapprove of surrogacy in any form.

There are at least five responses to surrogacy that a public body can have. First, it could remain neutral by doing nothing. Because of the involvement of third parties and potential conflict over rights, this option not reasonable. Second, if the public wants to encour-age surrogate motherhood, it could make surrogate contracts en-forceable and legally binding on all parties. No government body has recommended such an approach nor does there appear to be the least bit of sympathy for it. Regulation of surrogacy could be a third option. This could be accomplished by either limiting surrogacy to nonprofit-making agencies or by allowing profit-making agencies to practice but only within stringent controls and licensing. The Ontario Law Reform Commission recommendation of continuing involvement of a family law court to supervise the screening and counseling of the surrogate and client, review the contract, and monitor the surrogate fee is the only body that has taken this approach.

The fourth and fifth governmental options to commercial surrogacy are designed to limit its practice. One approach is to fail to recognize surrogate contracts as legitimate—to make them unenforceable as a matter of public policy. At the least, this has a chilling effect on commercial surrogacy, because since each party to the contract has to depend on the good faith of the other parties, this approach adds uncertainty to the whole process. This approach could be strengthened by making it clear that in custody disputes, the rights of the woman carrying the baby to term take precedence. In 1987, the Council of Europe's Ad Hoc Committee of Experts on Progress in the Biomedical Sciences (CAHBI), for example, stated that contracts for SM should be unenforceable and that intermediaries and advertising should be forbidden. In Germany, several courts have ruled SM contracts void, one concluding that the child's custody cannot be supplanted by a pre-birth agreement by the mother to surrender custody. Similarly, in Sweden, the Insemination Committee stated that SM is indefensible because of the risk of children becoming commodities.

The most drastic action to limit commercial surrogacy, and one which appears to be increasing in popularity, is prohibition. A 1985 resolution to the European Parliament condemned SM and encouraged member states to pass legislation making it a criminal offense. One of the first recommendations of the Warnock Commission acted upon by Parliament was passage of the Surrogate Arrangements Act (July 1985) which banned commercial surrogacy in the United Kingdom. Although this act does not outlaw payment of money by the couple or receipt of money by the SM, it does prohibit advertising as well as initiation or involvement in negotiations for a surrogacy arrangement or any contemplation of payment. Convictions under the act can result in fines up to 2000 pounds. In France, both agencies and individuals who use their services for SM arrangements are subject to prosecution. The French Ministry of Health recently dissolved three commercial surrogacy agencies, making them illegal.

In New South Wales, it is illegal under adoption laws for a mother giving up a baby to designate to whom it will go. In Victoria, commercial surrogacy is illegal under the Infertility (Medical Procedures) Act. Likewise, SM is illegal in Greece, the German Democratic Republic, and Denmark. The Health Council in Netherlands has recommended that commercial surrogacy be forbidden by law as has a recent report in Austria. Finally, the Commission for the Study of Human In Vitro Fertilization and Artificial Insemination in Spain (1986) recommended that all parties to a SM contract, including the lawyers, agencies, and physicians, should be subject to criminal penalties.

From this overview of legislation, regulations, committee recommendations, and court rulings across these many countries, it is obvious that commercial surrogacy has generated considerable opposition on public policy grounds. The direct inclusion of third parties with a clear financial stake, as well as the potential legal custody challenges that SM raises and the potential for commodifying children, has led to a cold reception for commercial surrogacy in virtually all countries that have faced the issue.

HUMAN EMBRYO RESEARCH

Certain to be one of the most volatile and sensitive set of issues surrounding human reproductive intervention centers on human embryo research. Explicit opposition comes from the right-to-life interests, who find research on embryos morally repugnant. Even persons who have no moral objections, however, have practical concerns for any research involving human material. Because the objectives of potential research range from increased knowledge of fertilization, understanding the causes of infertility and cancer, and treatment of genetic disease on the one hand to the creation of chimeras or clones and eugenic applications on the other, the issues are multifaceted and the debate intense. Support for some applications is often tempered with the need to devise mechanisms to control tightly what types of research are conducted. For instance, should consent of the genetic parents be necessary? More than other interventions discussed here which are clinical in nature, human embryo research has produced heated controversy in those countries that have attempted to deal with it. Despite vehement opposition from the Roman Catholic Church to any human embryo research, however, many European countries are moving toward legislation that permits research under strict limits (Dickson 1988:1117).

As a result of the politically explosive nature of embryo research, and to some extent because its ties to overcoming infertility are at best indirect, policy on it is less developed than AID, IVF, or SM. At least 23 jurisdictions (16 countries) have addressed the issue either through law, regulation, or commission reports (see table 6.2). Of these, about half currently allow research on spare embryos created for IVF, and most of these set a limit on research until 14 days after fertilization. There are, however, political moves in some of these countries to ban embryo research completely.

Even more controversial is the creation of human embryos solely for research purposes. This procedure cannot be defended on grounds that it simply makes use of embryos that would otherwise be destroyed; in addition, it raises the fears in some persons of a brave new world scenario of expediency or of a Nazi-type research mentality. Not surprisingly, only two jurisdictions (Ontario and Sweden) have endorsed the acceptability of producing human embryos specifically for research purposes, and both have recommended stringent regulation of the type of research to be conducted. The Ontario Law Reform Commission report of 1985 supported, in principle, research on both surplus and expressly created embryos to a 14–day limit. This conflicts with the 1984 recommendation of the Standing Committee on Ethics on Experimentation of the Medical Research Panel of Canada, which opposed the creation of embryos for research and limited spare embryo research to that which improves infertility management. Sweden's Committee on Genetic Integrity (1984) accepted research on embryos but recommended creation of strict guidelines including a strong medical foundation, donor consent for any research, and the prohibition of implantation and development in vivo of any embryos exposed to experiments. Any violation of these guidelines, they urged, should come under severe ethical examination.

On the other end of the spectrum, a 1987 law in Denmark bans all research on human embryos until a National Ethics Committee proposes to Parliament national guidelines for such research. Similarly, the Medical Council of Ireland, in 1985, approved guidelines that found human embryo experimentation unacceptable. Finally, in 1985, the Swiss Academy of Medical Sciences issued a directive that embryos should be kept alive only during the course of treatment—human embryo research should not be allowed. Later that year, however, a referendum called for the government to amend the federal constitution to allow regulation of research in human genetics and reproductive manipulation. A federal commission was created in 1986 to study the issue. Upon completion of the report and after consultation with all interested parties, a government opinion will be submitted to Parliament for consideration.

The subject of human embryo research continues to elicit considerable opposition in West Germany. The Benda report (1985) concluded that it is not justified to produce human embryos without the intent of implanting them. Research could be justifiable only if it assisted in diagnosing, preventing, or curing a disease of a specific embryo or if it led to specific medical findings of great value. The Joint Ministry of Justice and Ministry of Research and Technology Report (1985) concluded that embryo research was "harmful to human dignity."

In that context, the Ministry of Justice (1986) drafted legislation severely restricting such research, including penalties of up to five years imprisonment for engaging in embryo research without permission of the genetic parents. Also penalized under this draft legislation would be performance of IVF without the intent to implant the resulting embryos, maintenance of in vitro embryos past the point of normal implantation, artificial maintenance of nonviable embryos, and the creation of chimeras or clones. Despite an especially vocal outcry against these proposed restrictions from the German Medical Association and others, on grounds of scientific freedom and the "imperative" of human embryo research, a federal-state working group report published in 1987 concurred with the draft legislation that the creation of embryos for research purposes be a criminal offense. Also forbidden should be research on spare embryos, altering the genetic makeup of an individual, splitting embryos, creating chimeras, and cloning. According to Dickson (1988:1117), the "driving force behind the proposed legislation in Germany is a reawakening of national sensibilities over human experimentation carried out by Nazi doctors" and deeply held convictions about the status of early embryos as potential human beings.

Between those jurisdictions which support research on all available human embryos and those which reject such research fully, there are about ten countries that allow research only on "spare" embryos. In general, they tend to align with the 1987 principles laid down by the Council of Europe's Ad Hoc Committee of Experts

on Progress in the Biomedical Sciences which state that the creation of embryos for research purposes should be forbidden. Any
research that is allowed should benefit the embryo or at least do it
no harm. Moreover, if member countries allow such research, strict
conditions should be observed:

1. Research must have preventive, diagnostic, or therapeutic
   purposes for grave diseases of the embryo;
2. Other methods of achieving the purpose of the research must
   have been exhausted;
3. No embryo should be used later than 14 days after fertilization;
4. The consent of the genetic parents must be obtained; and
5. A multidisciplinary ethics committee must give prior approval to the research.

Even in many of these countries, however, the issue is far from
settled, as opposing interests have begun to enter the fray. There
are also evidences of disagreement between some states and their
national governments, leading to cross pressures for national government involvement.

In Australia, for instance, the Family Law Council Report (1985)
opposed all research on human embryos. In that same year, a bill
was proposed that would have prohibited any experimentation on
human embryos. Because of the heated controversy the bill created, it was referred to a senate select committee, the report of
which (*Human Embryo Experimentation in Australia*) was published
in 1986. In its report, the committee recommended that experiments designed as therapeutic for a specific embryo be allowed but
that all research resulting in destruction of the embryo be outlawed. The strong dissent to this recommendation assures continued debate. The committee also recommended an accreditation
and licensing system to assess every proposed experiment. Meanwhile, at the state level, Victoria and Western Australia allow embryo research. Although the 1984 Infertility (Medical Procedures)
Act in Victoria prohibits the production of embryos solely for research purposes, it permits research on spare embryos pending
prior approval of the specific experiment by the Standing Review
and Advisory Committee. Similarly, the 1986 report of the Committee to Enquire into the Social, Legal, and Ethical Issues relating
to In Vitro Fertilization in Western Australia found research on
surplus embryos acceptable.

Research on surplus human embryos has also been approved by committees in France (although it recommended a three-year moratorium on research aimed at making a genetic diagnosis prior to implantation) and Spain, where a parliamentary commission recommended that couples could donate embryos unused from IVF. Both bodies concluded that embryos should not be created solely for the purpose of research and that each experiment should be reviewed by an appropriate body. The Spanish Commission also requires permission of the genetic parents and proof that the research has positive goals for individuals or society. Furthermore, proposed law (122AE1000061) in Spain prohibits the buying and selling of human embryos or organs and prevents the conception or abortion of an embryo solely for purposes of tissue donation (Gracia, 1988:29). Regulations adopted in Israel in 1987 permit egg retrieval only for purposes of fertilization and implantation, thus effectively banning the production of embryos for research purposes, although it is unclear whether couples could donate surplus embryos, as in Spain and France.

In Austria, a 1986 report of the Ministry of Science and Research stated that research should be performed only on embryos that have no hope of implantation. Like that in several other jurisdictions, research in Austria requires approval from a local institutional review board, prior exhaustion of analogous animal research, the goal of prevention or cure of disease, no creation of humans with special characteristics, clones, chimeras, or hybrids. Similarly, the Health Council of the Netherlands stated that pre-embryo research is acceptable provided, among other things, that the data could not be obtained by different means, both genetic parents have given their consent, and the research is approved by a national committee. The Health Council also recommended that the legal status of the preimplantation embryo, the authority over the embryo by its genetic parents, and the functioning of embryo banks be regulated by law and that selling embryos should be outlawed.

In no country has there been more activity than Britain. In a strongly divided decision, the majority of the Warnock Committee recommended that research on embryos be allowed up to fourteen days after fertilization but only under license, with consent of the genetic parents when possible. Three of the sixteen members were opposed to all embryo research, while four others opposed experimentation on embryos created solely for the purpose of research.

The committee also recommended that the government create a statutory licensing authority (SLA) to regulate such research. The Voluntary Licensing Authority (VLA) was established by the Medical Research Council and Royal College of Obstetricians and Gynaecologists in 1986 as an interim measure until the government acted.

The Government White Paper issued in November 1987, however, did not follow the recommendations of the Warnock Committee nor the interim guidelines. The government proposed criminal offenses for research on genetic manipulation of human embryos, the cloning of embryos, or the creation of hybrid embryos. It also left two alternatives to embryo research to a Parliament "free vote" which allows members to vote their conscience. The first option is a complete prohibition of such research except where there is an intention to transfer the embryos to a gestational mother as part of an IVF procedure. The second option, the one recommended by the Warnock Committee and reflective of the Council of Europe's principles, allows controlled research on embryos up to fourteen days after fertilization to be carried out under the auspices of an independent SLA. Under this alternative, the SLA would be empowered to license scientists and physicians performing embryo research or IVF and would make decisions based on the scientific validity of the research, its purpose of advancing diagnostic or therapeutic techniques of fertility control, the absence of reasonable research alternatives, and the informed consent of the gamete or embryo donors. Whatever decision Parliament ultimately makes will be highly controversial.

The experience of these countries on the thorny issues of embryo research illustrates the difficulty of resolving them. This brief overview of activity, however, shows that at least several other countries are ahead of the U.S. in terms of facing the issues. The moratorium on NIH funding of embryo research since 1980 and the logjam in Congress on this issue has limited public dialogue at a time when other countries are establishing policy.

This discussion also demonstrates how complex this issue is and what some of the policy options are. In addition to the broad questions of whether embryo research should be allowed, and, if so, whether embryos can be produced specifically for research purposes, are more subtle issues over the role of genetic parents, the commodification of embryos, and the best mechanisms for regulating such research. It also raises practical questions concerning the extent to which limiting research to spare or surplus embryos from IVF will inhibit critical research on the one hand, and lead to increased pressures to produce more "spare" embryos through superovulation on the other. Any meaningful effort by U.S. policy makers to regulate human embryo research should consider the activities of other countries outlined here. Finally, this discussion again shows that these issues are cross-national in scope and that closing down embryo research in some countries might be of limited significance if other countries allow it. Unlike AID and IVF, where an international consensus is growing, embryo research is considerably more complicated.

CONCLUSIONS

Despite the wide variation in the mode and comprehensiveness of the responses of these countries to the issues surrounding reproductive technologies, several international patterns are emerging. Basically, AIH and AID have gained widespread acceptance by policy makers and ethics committees. In most countries, the child of AID with the husband's consent is considered irrefutably a legitimate offspring of the husband. Similarly, IVF is widely accepted if it is conducted on married (or stable) couples and donor eggs are not used. IVF has less support when donor gametes are used, however, and almost none for use by singles. Most countries also realize the need for some type of regulation of AID and IVF facilities, although action to that end is fragmented to date.

In contrast, surrogate motherhood, especially commercial surrogacy, has been rejected by virtually every country which has considered it. With only several exceptions, surrogacy contracts are either unenforceable or illegal. There is considerable sympathy for the imposition of criminal penalties on agencies that practice surrogacy for a profit. Interestingly, there has been very little debate in these countries over the issue of payment to surrogate mothers, which has monopolized much of the discussion in the U.S. In large part, payment has not been at issue, probably because it need not be if SM is not allowed at all.

Finally, the controversy over research on human embryos appears to be similar across all countries and largely reflects the expression of it in the U.S. Although over half of these jurisdictions presently allow research on surplus embryos, there are indications that tighter restrictions are inevitable in many of these countries because of pressures from mobilizing groups. More objectionable is the production of embryos specifically for research purposes. There is little backing for this practice in evidence in the reports of the major bodies that have studied it, despite substantial testimony from the scientific community that it is needed to ensure an adequate supply of embryos for critical medical research.

The most important contribution of the myriad of comparative policy activity on reproductive technologies, however, is to illustrate the range of mechanisms available to deal with the issues they raise. It is striking that the U.S. did not have any single body on the scale of the Warnock Committee in Britain or the Waller Commission in Victoria. In part, this neglect is a function of our pluralist, federal system and the lack of a clear agenda-setting role of the government that is present in a parliamentary system. It also reflects the fact that these technologies have largely been placed in an individual rights context in the U.S. where governmental involvement is viewed as a threat, not protection, of the individual. This, in combination with the tendency of the Reagan and Bush Administrations and Congress to steer clear of these issues for political reasons, have retarded the national dialogue until very recently. The result is a need to move quickly on these issues. To that end, the experiences of the countries discussed here should serve as valuable lessons in determining how best to regulate reproduction.

CHAPTER SEVEN

The National Policy Context: Options and Problems

I CONCLUDED chapter 5 by arguing that while the recent interest in TMR of some state legislatures is welcome but overdue, and while the standards promulgated by professional associations are laudable, adequate regulation of these technologies requires action at the national level. The high economic stakes, the resulting trend toward commercialization, and the continuing questions of access to, and equity of, these services reinforces the need for a national perspective to regulating reproductive services. Chapter 6 described attempts by other countries to provide coordinated national policies on TMR and demonstrated certain patterns that were emerging that might be useful in formulating a national policy in the United States.

At a more conceptual level, the issues raised by TMR, especially as they relate to women and minorities who are vulnerable to

169

potential abuse and to the children who are unwitting products of
the techniques, must be exposed to broader public scrutiny. Cumulatively, these technologies do represent a revolution that challenges basic social values and existing social structures. As such,
they necessitate a change in the way we think about ourselves, our
children, and our responsibilities to future generations. These issues raise formidable policy questions of the proper role of government in human reproduction, the most effective means of government involvement, the appropriate mechanisms for setting social
priorities, and ultimately, who decides and controls the use of
genetic and reproductive technologies in a democratic society. At
the most abstract level, these technologies return us to basic philosophical questions that have long framed western political thought
concerning the meaning of human existence, the relationship of the
individual to the state, and the immutability of human nature.

This chapter addresses the issues relating to the role of government in dealing with the social problems that accompany the revolution in human reproduction. After describing the range of policy
options and the potential levels of government involvement, attention is directed to the unique characteristics of the existing U.S.
political system that frame the boundaries of government action
and, I argue, inhibit the capacity to develop adequate policy responses. The critical issue of the extent to which the public should
participate in decision-making regarding technologies that hold
considerable personal, as well as social, importance is analyzed
within a broader discussion of democracy in a technological era.

PUBLIC POLICY OPTIONS

The policy problems raised by reproductive technology are among
the most volatile and incisive issues imaginable. They do not fit the
traditional mold of political issues that are resolved through a
bargaining and compromise process. Instead, they demonstrate
fundamental value conflicts over meanings of human life and death,
which themselves reflect basic tenets of a variety of religious and
secular ethical frameworks. Societies do not often debate fundamental definitions, but when they do, volatility results. Moreover,
the rapid pace of technological change has created these value
conflicts over a very short time span, whereas values themselves
normally change gradually over generations through a socializa-

tion process. Although there is no doubt that these issues are difficult to deal with politically, thereby explaining the tendency of
many officials to avoid them when possible, the rapid advances in
technology make it mandatory that action be taken—at least to
discuss the issues—within the political context.

Every government has at its disposal an array of policy options
to deal with the problems raised by reproductive technology. One
option, which until now has been the option of choice for many
policy makers in the U.S., is to take no action on the basis that it is
a matter of private, not public, concern. Given the developments
discussed earlier, however, this approach is not adequate. No longer
can decision makers abdicate the responsibility to face the societal
ramifications of human genetic and reproductive technologies.

Once the government becomes actively involved in the issues of
reproductive technologies, many other options are possible. Although the details of specific policy responses are unbounded in
variety, the general categories of action can be classified on a
continuum with prohibition on one extreme and mandate on the
other (figure 7.1). In between is an array of regulatory and distrib-
utive policies that can serve to either encourage or discourage
development and use of the technologies. Although it is likely that
the most feasible and effective forms of government intervention
will be the latter—more moderate—ones, considerable debate in
the literature has focused on the most intrusive—prohibition and
mandate—types.

The most straightforward form of prohibition is to create laws
that impose criminal sanctions on a particular activity. One recent
example of this approach is the Michigan statute that bans commercial surrogacy. Other examples are state laws that prohibit
research on human embryos or the use of fetal tissue. Opponents of
prohibition of research often argue that such action represents
infringement of First Amendment rights and of scientific freedom
of inquiry. Another more practical objection is that by banning

---

FIGURE 7.1. Types of Government Involvement in Human Genetics
and Reproduction

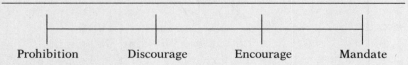

| Prohibition | Discourage | Encourage | Mandate |

certain categories of research in the U.S. or in one state, it will simply be moved elsewhere; perhaps without the kind of protections that could be imposed, short of prohibition. Proponents of prohibition argue that protection of some broader public interest or the interests of vulnerable individuals requires proscribing such research.

Prohibiting the use of reproductive technologies by individuals is even more problematic because it may conflict with constitutional law rulings that have given special protection to the procreative autonomy of individuals. According to Dresser (1985:167), infertile couples could challenge successfully a governmental ban as an unjust interference with a fundamental right, unless the government could demonstrate a compelling state interest. The laws prohibiting SM, for instance, will have to withstand constitutional challenges by demonstrating that they prevent harm to any of the parties to the contract or to the offspring. Also, outlawing use of a technique is unlikely to be effective if it is legal in other jurisdictions. For example, if Ohio permits SM, the Michigan ban might simply become a discriminatory policy against those persons unable to arrange for a surrogacy across the state line. Similarly, attempts by the U.S. government to ban the sale or use of RU486 (a drug that induces abortion) are likely to prove futile if there is a strong public demand and it is available in other countries.

Another common use of the term prohibition in the U.S. refers to a ban on government funding of a certain line of research. This can be a very effective means of control over research priorities where there is little motivation by the private sphere to fund it. Because of the commercial attractiveness of many reproductive applications, however, prohibiting government funding no longer ensures that the research will stop. Ironically, what this does is to force such research outside the peer review process needed for governmental sponsorship, effectively negating this means of control and monitoring. It could lead to less control over the research in the long run, because of the development of a large private research establishment. To a large extent, this scenario has been played out with IVF and other TMRs in light of the de facto moratorium on federal funding of human embryo and fetal research over the last decade, due to the abolition of the Ethics Advisory Board.

Another practical limitation in prohibiting the funding of targeted categories of research derives from the lack of clear-cut lines of demarcation in basic research. For instance, a substantial proportion of the basic research leading to human applications is directed instead at animal breeding and, to a lesser extent, agriculture. Furthermore, human reproductive and genetic techniques often are made possible because of knowledge gained in other areas of basic biological or medical research. Restraining potential research advances leading to human egg fusion and cloning, for example, would preclude certain areas of cancer and AIDS research. Banning certain lines of reproductive research, in turn, carries with it the probability of inhibiting a considerably broader range of benefits that might follow. These interrelationships across diverse areas of basic research serve to complicate considerably the question of public control.

The other extreme of policy reaction to human reproductive technologies is to mandate the use of particular techniques. The clearest examples of mandatory legislation regarding human reproduction are the eugenic sterilization laws that many states implemented earlier in this century. More recent examples are the mandatory sickle-cell screening statutes in Massachusetts and other states in the early 1970s and the laws requiring screening of all newborns for phenylketonuria (PKU) in at least 43 states. The development of accurate DNA probes for a variety of conditions, including susceptibility to workplace hazards, could lead to renewed calls for mandated genetic screening programs.

Finally, some courts have ordered women to undergo caesarean sections against their will, for the benefit of their babies (Nelson and Millikin 1988). Could this be extended to mandated invasions of the mother's body to allow surgery on the fetus in utero? Or could states mandate collaborative procreation for individuals who are identified as carrying deleterious genes such as that for Huntington's disease? In other words, could these individuals be required to use other persons' germ materials if they choose to have children? Given our constitutional framework, it is unlikely that such programs would be upheld by the courts, even if enacted by the legislatures. It is more likely that measures short of mandate will be enacted to foster use of applications deemed to be in the public interest. As is evident by the use of a continuum rather than discrete categories, however, the line between mandate and encouragement is a cloudy one.

The government has at its disposal an arsenal of means to encourage the use of reproduction technology. The primary means, of course, are financial. Vigorous funding of particular research places a high social priority on that area and draws researchers toward it. Moreover, once an area of research becomes established, it tends to generate its own momentum. Public funding is also a factor in encouraging individual use of technologies once they are available. The provision of publicly supported prenatal testing programs expands the use of amniocentesis and other techniques. Public funding of genetic screening programs, combined with programs designed to educate the public on the availability and use of these services, also heightens use. And, certainly, public support programs for IVF and other infertility treatments will encourage the proliferation of such services. In addition to the provision of public services and education programs, the government can enhance use through tax incentives either to the users, or to the providers, of these services.

Although the primary goal of many of these government programs is equity of access to services, they do tend to encourage use. The long and bitter battle over public funding of abortions demonstrates how intense the reactions to this reality are when an interest is opposed to the technique. From the other end of the political spectrum, some feminist and handicapped advocacy groups are adamantly opposed to public funding of sterilization, which they contend leads to abuse. While means to encourage use are less controversial than clear government mandates for use, they engender considerable opposition under some circumstances.

The government can also discourage use of techniques through several approaches. First, it can do so by withholding public funding for a particular service. To a large extent this has been the reaction to TMRs of most U.S. jurisdictions until this time. In the area of reproduction, however, this tactic raises questions of equity on a fundamental right. The exclusion of public funding means that those persons without adequate resources for access to the technologies cannot exercise a Court-defined right to privacy in procreation. This form of discouragement is, therefore, discriminatory, because it has that function only for persons who lack either adequate personal resources or private third-party coverage.

A second way of discouraging the use of techniques is for the state to fail to provide legal protection to the parties involved. For instance, short of banning commercial surrogacy, many states are moving toward making surrogate contracts unenforceable or void, thus making the practice very risky for the participants, particularly the couple who puts up the money. Likewise, in those jurisdictions where a sperm donor is not explicitly given legal protection against paternity of the AID child, or conversely, the couple is not given assurances that the husband is the legal father, AID becomes more problematic.

The third, and possibly most effective, approach to deterring the provision and, therefore, the use of reproductive technologies is through the powers of states to protect the public health. The states regulate most private health agents through licensing requirements. So far, TMR services have escaped licensing controls applied to most other areas of public life including restaurants, bars, and hotels. The states, however, do have it within their power to set licensing criteria which require that IVF centers meet certain minimal standards regarding the skills and knowledge of personnel. Moreover, application of certificate-of-need legislation could enable the government to set limits in the number of such facilities. As evidenced by recent legislation in several states, the government has the power to regulate the payment of fees for particular services. States, then, could clearly discourage the private sector from offering new reproductive technologies by imposing burdensome regulatory requirements and exorbitant licensing fees (Dresser 1985:167). Except for SM, however, there has been little movement by the states to take even minimal licensing action to regulate these technologies. Any such attempts, of course, would have to be justified by demonstrating that the regulations were necessary to protect the public health or some other vital state interest.

As with prohibition, regulation in the U.S. often refers only to those activities funded by public dollars. For instance, the recombinant DNA regulations imposed by the federal government in 1976 never legally applied to privately funded research, although most private researchers found it in their interests to comply voluntarily. The federal government also has broad powers to regulate interstate commerce. It is possible that some reproductive services could be exempt, but it is likely that most would come under the control of interstate commerce as broadly defined by the courts. The Federal Trade Commission and Federal Communications Commission would also likely have the power to regulate the marketing of TMRs by private enterprises.

Each of the policy options—prohibition, mandate, encouragement, and regulation—raises constitutional, social, and political questions. Moreover, to complicate matters, for each of these policy options, there are three distinct policy areas that are critical to reproductive technologies. Policy might be made regarding: (1) research and development of particular technologies; (2) their availability, accessibility, and use by individuals; and (3) their aggregate social consequences. Because the basic research leading to reproductive technology is dependent on federal funding, research and development is, at least theoretically, influenced at the national level. If the research has a well-determined economic payoff, however, the funding strategy must be supplemented by regulation, because private industry operates independently of the guidelines for receiving governmental support. Rather than elaborating the government's potential role in precluding certain basic research and technological development, it is more reasonable to stress the government's ability to define research priorities through its funding policies. The assumption here is that the timing of the future availability of a specific reproductive innovation can be influenced, though the international nature of reproductive research proscribes rigid national control over technology.

In addition to influencing the development of reproductive technologies, the government might become involved in the individual or aggregate use of these techniques. The most likely forms such intervention might take include encouragement of use by provision of free services, education programs, or financial inducements, or, conversely, discouragement of use by reducing accessibility or imposing direct controls. Also, consumer protection and regulation of the marketing of TMRs can influence individual use. At the extremes, individual use of specific reproductive technologies might be mandated or prohibited. The range of options available to the government to intervene in the procreative process is vast, and, despite cultural predispositions toward individual reproductive choice in the United States, many policy controversies center on questions of the proper role of the government involving individual applications.

The third level of policy concern is directed toward the aggregate social consequences of these technologies, both singly and cumulatively. Although one might argue that individuals must judge for themselves how a specific technology will affect them, the use of a technique such as sex preselection, by large numbers of people over time, could have severe consequences for society as a whole, especially future generations. Also, the cumulative impact of all intervention techniques has the potential to alter drastically social values and structures at the base of our society. A critical policy question, then, is what role does the government have in assessing the social consequences of reproductive technologies and in controlling the use of these techniques to protect the long-term public interest?

On the one hand, because many aspects of these issues are matters of private judgment not requiring collective decisions, they ought to be left as much as possible to the individuals affected. Moreover, because of our pluralistic tradition, the more devolution possible—for example, to institutional review boards, to hospitals, to physicians and patients—the better. In contrast, it seems that, at the least, the government has a duty in its role of the protector of public health to define national goals and provide the mechanisms by which priorities for society can be established. Assuming a continuing context of scarce resources, there is considerable need for: (1) extensive data to predict possible consequences of alternative courses of action; (2) mechanisms to provide accurate means of monitoring on a continuous basis consequences of the actions taken; and (3) strategies for coping with consequences judged undesirable. Of all social institutions, only the government has the capacity to accomplish these multiple purposes, and then only with considerable commitment and effort.

Although policy making at each of these three levels might appear distinctive, all three are linked together inextricably, because priorities set at an early stage of research will directly influence later applications. Moreover, policies aimed at ameliorating the adverse consequences of widespread use of reproductive technologies in society necessarily affect intervention at the individual level. In turn, encouraging or preempting individual usage of a specific technique will be felt in the research community, as demands for particular services increase or decline. Any comprehensive policy, therefore, must address problems in all three areas. Not surprisingly, there is significant controversy over whether the government should be involved at any stage in the development and application of reproductive technologies. Some observers contend that the government should have no role in reproductive choice, no matter how it is implemented, while others see an important positive role at one or all of the levels discussed above. Figure 7.2 arrays a variety of positions regarding government activity in human reproduction. In this figure, two continuums are presented: support or opposition for reproductive technologies and support or opposition for government intervention. The figure does not distinguish between those who favor a government role in research and those who approve of intervention in use either by individuals or in the aggregate.

A close reading of figure 7.2 demonstrates that there is little clarity over what government involvement entails. In their arguments, opponents and proponents of public action tend to emphasize the policy options which best fit their goals and ignore the others. Moreover, those persons who favor the technologies emphasize public funding of research and development of programs designed to encourage usage, while those opposed to the technologies include persons who want the government to prohibit certain areas of research, or those who want the government to stay out of genetic and reproductive research and application out of a fear of potential social-control policy (Chorover 1980). Figure 7.2 also indicates that the policy debate will continue to be most volatile concerning mandated programs, as some of the most adamant proponents of technology favor such programs on grounds of public health or eugenics, while those of a variety of persuasions fear that government involvement will lead to a brave new world of social control over reproduction or represent threats to strongly held beliefs.

Figure 7.2 illustrates, however, that government involvement of some form appears essential to most proponents and opponents of specific reproductive technologies. Even the few viewpoints located on the right side of the figure imply a limited government role. At a minimum, those in quadrant II want some governmental protection of the right to free individual procreative choice, while those in quadrant IV demand adequate social mechanisms to ensure that technologies are not directed toward eugenic or social control ends. As noted earlier, the most obvious institutions for realizing these goals in a democracy are public institutions. The momentum of reproductive and genetic technology is too strong to channel, without an active public involvement at the national level.

CONSTRAINTS ON ACTION IN THE UNITED STATES POLITICAL SYSTEM

Despite the urgent need for concerted action at the national level to establish a balanced and workable framework for dealing with

FIGURE 7.2. The Role of Government in Reproductive Choice

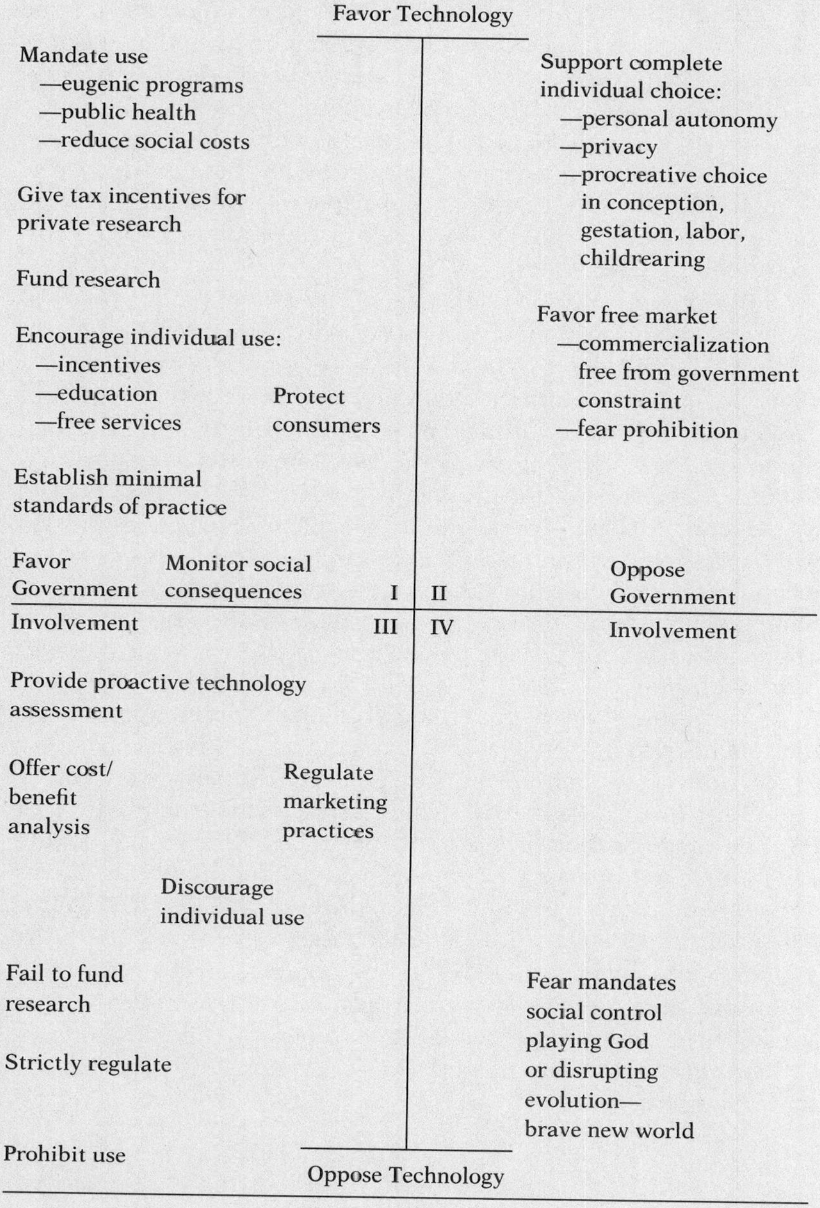

Favor Technology

Mandate use
  —eugenic programs
  —public health
  —reduce social costs

Give tax incentives for
private research

Fund research

Encourage individual use:
  —incentives
  —education   Protect
  —free services   consumers

Establish minimal
standards of practice

Favor   Monitor social   Oppose
Government   consequences   I | II   Government
Involvement   III | IV   Involvement

Provide proactive technology
assessment

Offer cost/   Regulate
benefit   marketing
analysis   practices

            Discourage
            individual use

Fail to fund   Fear mandates
research   social control
                                  playing God
Strictly regulate   or disrupting
                                  evolution—
                                  brave new world
Prohibit use

Support complete
individual choice:
  —personal autonomy
  —privacy
  —procreative choice
    in conception,
    gestation, labor,
    childrearing

Favor free market
  —commercialization
    free from government
    constraint
  —fear prohibition

Oppose Technology

the issues created by these burgeoning technologies, to date there
has been little activity by the federal government. To understand
why the United States trails other western countries in reacting to
the reproductive revolution, it is critical to examine the unique
characteristics of the U.S. political system. In fact, these factors
raise serious questions about the capacity of existing institutions
to deal with these emerging issues. William Carey (1982:2), for
instance, expresses little confidence in the ability of "our national
policy machinery" to recognize and deal with these policy issues.
He questions society's institutional capacities to formulate and
manage "strategies aimed toward modifying or altering future outcomes of near term issues."

One intrinsic characteristic pervading the American political
system is the dispersion of power throughout a variety of institutions. Although federalism and separation of powers have served a
valuable function by ensuring that no single branch of government
or agency monopolizes political power, the resulting fragmentation
of the system works counter to the development of long-term national policy. Instead, this fragmented policy-making process and
its tendency to focus on immediate, conspicuous problems has led
to a failure to provide systematic, comprehensive assessment of the
technologies or their implications for society. In contrast, the parliamentary systems of countries such as Britain permit a more
centralized basis for making policy, even on divisive issues such as
reproduction.

An accompanying characteristic of the U. S. political process is
the tendency to postpone action until the situation reaches crisis
proportions. It is doubtful that reproductive technology at present
represents a crisis, but it is clear that we cannot afford to wait
until such a situation develops. At that stage, it might be too late
to establish a framework for the rational deliberation of the issues
and resolution of the problems. Also, the extent to which the political institutions start a dialogue on these issues now, when the
technologies are in relatively early stages of development, will
determine their ability to react to future innovations destined to be
substantially more controversial. Consequently, this section criti-
cally examines the capacity of the major governmental institutions
to deal with reproductive issues.

The Courts

Much of the government activity regarding issues of reproduction continues to be found in the courts. Table 7.1 presents a view of the scope of judicial involvement. Despite the significant policy ramifications of court rulings, debate continues as to whether the courts ought to be involved in, or are capable of, a policy-making role. Critics (see Schoenberg 1979) charge that inherent limitations on judicial policy-making preclude an active role. Because the judicial process is passive and retrospective, it is viewed as too slow to react to rapid technological progress. Elliot L. Segall, president of the American Society of Law and Medicine, is quoted by Arehart-Treichel (1980:156) as contending that the "U.S. legal system is one generation behind medical science."

Also, because the primary function of the courts is to resolve conflicts centering on the rights and obligations of the parties before them, individual cases supposedly are decided on evidence produced by the parties to each case, not on grounds of public policy considerations. Although particular decisions might offer implicit principles with important policy implications, the courts "generally refrain from deciding individual cases on the basis of deliberately establishing public-policy controls" (Green 1976:171). In those instances where judicial decisions have consequences beyond the immediate parties to the case, there often are "serious difficulties in communicating new legal requirements to populations that are not yet within the jurisdiction of courts" (Nakamura and Smallwood 1980:107). As a result, decisions are episodic, unpredictable, and often inconsistent. Case-by-case adjudication across a wide variety of state and federal courts adds to the confusion. Due to the slowness of this process, it is not likely that we can rely on the courts to protect society against rapid technological developments.

In spite of the apparent limitations of the courts, they are at this stage unmistakably involved in the resolution of questions relating to individual use of reproductive technologies. One need only look at the broad impact of *Roe v. Wade,* or wrongful birth torts and the pressures they exert on physicians to utilize prenatal diagnostic techniques, to see social consequences extending beyond the original litigation. The expanding concept of fundamental rights, especially as it relates to privacy and self-determination in reproductive matters, and the notion of "compelling state interest" plainly demonstrate the practical influence of the courts on the application of reproductive technology. Despite the clear evidence that the

---

TABLE 7.1. Selected Areas of Judicial Involvement
in Reproduction

Preconception Torts
    Sterilization (consent questions)
    Contraception (accessibility)
    Medical malpractice
    Product liability
    Radiation injuries
    Workplace hazards
    Agent Orange cases

Wrongful Conception and Wrongful Pregnancy
    Failed sterilization
    Failed contraception
    Misdiagnosis or failure to diagnose pregnancy
    Unsuccessful abortion

Conception Stage
    Artificial insemination
    In vitro fertilization
    Embryo transfer
    Cryopreservation
    Surrogate motherhood

Prenatal Stage
    Abortion (accessibility, age, and other qualifications)
    Viability question
    Harm to fetus (mother, third parties)
    Fetus as patient
    Forced caesarian sections
    Fetus as organ or tissue supply

Neonatal Stage
    Intensive care (Baby Jane Doe, etc.)
    Neonatal euthanasia
    Torts for wrongful birth
    Torts for wrongful life

---

courts by default are being cast into these policy issues, it is not likely that they are either capable of, or willing to play, a critical role in setting societal priorities and goals regarding re productive technology or in assessing their social consequences in any systematic manner. For resolution of those broader social issues, attention must be turned toward administrative agencies and Congress.

Congress

Although Congress bears primary responsibility for lawmaking un-der the Constitution, it is not well suited for making policy on issues as elaborate as human reproduction. As a deliberative body, Congress is extremely slow—both in recognizing policy problems and in acting upon them. According to Shick (1977:10), the "legis-lative process is weighted against quick and comprehensive re-sponses" and encourages negotiation and compromise to build ma-jorities at each stage. The issues raised by reproductive technology, however, are qualitatively different from traditional public issues which revolve around expenditures of funds. Although reproduc-tive issues include that dimension, they also encompass difficult moral aspects that legislatures try to avoid. As stated by Joseph Coates (1978:33), "cut and fit accommodation and incremental change, the traditional strategies of government, are increasingly ineffective, if not sterile modes of operation."

Reinforcing this inherent congressional bias against quick and comprehensive response to problems is a tendency of Congress to refrain from enacting regulatory laws until there is an obvious need for legislation. Because Congress is too busy with urgent problems, it fails to direct adequate attention to less pressing is-sues. This orientation results in a circular pattern of priority set-ting that is difficult to alter, because the practice of ignoring prob-lems until they become critical leaves little time to deal with anything but immediate problems. This pattern makes it improba-ble that Congress as currently structured can be depended on to assess and evaluate policy issues that are more remote. Also, con-gressmen seldom win reelection on the basis of their involvement in future-oriented legislation.

Congress also distinctly demonstrates the fragmentation of power in U.S. institutions. Although the rationale behind the committee system is to divide labor and thereby maximize skill and minimize the overall workload, Tribe (1973:609) concludes that "the existing system of specialized committees, riddled with rivalries and fragmented by jurisdictional division, cannot be relied upon to provide the focus without which public concern is just so much undirected energy." The present committee system fails to reflect cross-cutting issues and increases duplication as numerous committees stake claims to jurisdiction on important issues. This further slows the process without assurance that relevant policy interdependencies will be considered. Since reproductive issues tend to combine what in the past were perceived to be separate issues and have multiplied the number of interests to be considered, the process is frustrated.

Specialization in Congress has also led to a situation where few members are well informed about any specific issue. Voting is often the product of cue-giving by those colleagues considered substantive experts, or the result of logrolling or vote tradeoffs. Seldom are more than a handful of members familiar with any piece of technical legislation. Schoenberg (1979:93) concludes that "legislators are frequently unsophisticated about science and do not understand the fundamental issues involved in the application of new discoveries." Hearings are characterized by low attendance, and congressmen tend to be responsive to selective testimony, often from those who have a high stake on either side of the issue. As an example, when the Subcommittee on Regulation and Business Opportunities of the House Committee on Small Business held hearings (U.S. Congress 1988) on the vital issue of consumer protection involving IVF clinics, of the 13 members only the Subcommittee chairman was in attendance.

Despite the failure of Congress to enact legislation, it is far from oblivious to the policy issues surrounding reproductive technologies. The Office of Technology Assessment (OTA), created by Congress in 1972 to provide analytical studies and advice, has issued a series of important reports on infertility, gene mapping, artificial insemination, and workplace screening. These studies, each requested by members of Congress or by congressional committees, include discussions of policy options as well as the legal and social dimensions. Although the recency of these studies precludes the criticism that they have yet to result in substantive action by Congress, based on the response to other OTA reports one can not be overly optimistic. Hopefully, the study on infertility (OTA 1988) will lead at least to heightened awareness of the issues on Capital Hill.

Notwithstanding recent hearings (see chapter 5), Congress continues to shy away from the issue of human reproduction. For reasons cited above, most elected officials have little to gain by entering the debate over reproductive choice, nor do they have the technical background necessary to deliberate on the advisibility of the many technological applications. Also, despite attempts by conservative congressmen to outlaw embryo and fetal research and by others to tighten control of biomedical research by reassessing the role of Congress in the National Institutes of Health (NIH) and the National Science Foundation (NSF), as a body, Congress seems willing to allow wide discretion to the administrative agencies rather than enter the controversy and establish a national reproductive policy. Given the current political climate and the volatile nature of reproductive issues, such inaction should come as no surprise.

The Federal Bureaucracy

The massive scope and complexity of the federal bureaucracy, combined with its fragmented jurisdictional boundaries, have resulted in overlapping and confusing lines of authority. Nowhere is this more obvious than in reproductive policy. The following is a list of some of the federal agencies involved in either reproductive research or application.

A. Health Care Financing Administration (Health Standards and Quality Bureau)
B. Public Health Service
  1. Centers for Disease Control (Center for Health Promotion and Education, Division of Reproductive Health)
  2. Food and Drug Administration
    a. Center for Drugs and Biologics (Office of Biologics Research and Review, Office of Compliance)
    b. Center for Devices and Radiological Health (Office of Device Evaluation, Office of Compliance, Office of Science and Technology)
  3. Health Resources and Services Administration (Bureau of

Health Care Delivery and Assistance, Division of Maternal and Child Health)
4. National Center for Health Services Research (Office of Health Technology Assessment)
5. National Institutes of Health
   a. National Institute of Child Health and Human Development
      - Center for Population Research (Reproductive Sciences Branch)
      - Center for Research for Mothers and Children
      - Intramural Research Program (Human Genetics Branch, Endocrinology and Reproduction Research)
   b. National Institute of General Medical Services (Genetics Program)
   c. Division of Research Resources
C. Consumer Product Safety Commission
D. National Science Foundation
E. Veterans Administration

Given the development of these agencies and their competition for influence or even survival, there is nothing approaching a single locus of power for reproductive policy making. There is no coordinating mechanism to ensure that policy is consistent or to eliminate the duplication and confusion that result with numerous agencies making policy in the same substantive area. Another unfortunate byproduct of these overlapping jurisdictions is that agencies do not always cooperate fully with each other. Comprehensive and future-oriented policy is unlikely as long as this competition exists.

A problem inherent to bureaucracies, which minimizes their objectivity and causes them to lose sight of broader public responsibilities, is their dependence on special interest group support. Even though the demands on each agency are likely to be diverse, as stakeholders maneuver to influence policy decisions, agencies are cognizant of the need to maintain mutually beneficial relationships with their clients. As a result, "the larger diffuse goals of public interest easily become contracted to mean the goals of self-interested clients who are organized, constantly on the job defining problems, providing information and seeking advantage" (Freeman 1974:160). Among the national groups actively involved in reproductive policy matters are:

Alan Guttmacher Institute
Alternatives to Abortion International
American College of Obstetricians and Gynecologists
American Fertility Society
American Medical Association
American Public Health Association
Americans United for Life
Association for Voluntary Surgical Contraception
Association of Reproductive Health Professionals
Catholics for a Free Choice
Coalition for the Medical Rights of Women
Committee for Responsible Genetics
Committee to Defend Reproductive Rights
Federation of Organizations of Professional Women
Fertility Research Foundation
Lesbian Rights Project
National Abortion Federation
National Abortion Rights Action League
National Association of Surrogate Mothers
National Clearinghouse for Family Planning Information
National Council of Churches
National Family Planning and Reproductive Health Association, Inc.
National Genetics Foundation
National Organization for Women
National Research Foundation for Fertility
National Women's Health Network
Planned Parenthood Federation of America, Inc.
Religious Coalition for Abortion Rights
Reproductive Freedom Project—ACLU
RESOLVE, Inc.
The National Foundation—March of Dimes
Society of Assisted Reproductive Technology
Synagogue Council of America
U.S. Catholic Conference

Given the paramount role of special interests in the existing bureaucratic system and the fragmentation across the agencies, it seems that if the government is to make objective and comprehensive reproductive policy, an agency must be created which is free from domination by interest groups while it allows for widespread public access. This appears unlikely, however, within the current institutional context where the growth and survival of a public agency depends upon its success in establishing routinized relationships with its clients. Like Congress, the bureaucracy, at least as it now operates, appears incapable of dealing with complex and controversial problems raised by reproductive technologies.

Ad hoc Mechanisms

National commissions, advisory councils, and other temporary mechanisms traditionally have been created when specific problems have reached national attention or when public officials feel that creation of such bodies is politically warranted. These ad hoc mechanisms often serve to buy time for the officials until the problem becomes less salient. By calling for and establishing a commission in response to a crisis instead of introducing legislation directly, the decision maker might be able to defuse an otherwise explosive situation and reduce public pressure for immediate action. Moreover, commissions have the capability of functioning outside the glare of publicity and present an image of impartiality.

Because all findings of commissions are advisory only, they are not binding at any stage in the policy process. They can only recommend. Furthermore, the dissemination of the final report depends not on the quality of the report, but on how it corresponds to the perceptions of the officials who commissioned it. In other words, the ultimate influence of these advising mechanisms depends on how well their findings are received by those in authority. Also, because their tenure is specified by statute and usually limited to four years or less, commissions cannot provide continuous review and evaluation. Although these mechanisms serve a valuable service by raising issues, demonstrating complex interrelationships, and setting the boundaries for debate, they seldom offer continued scrutiny of the issue. Since reproductive technology is advancing at a rapid rate, even the definitions of problems are temporary and subject to change with the next technological development. Despite these limitations, it is expected that much of the effort to deal with human reproductive issues will be, initially at least, delegated to ad hoc commissions as it already has been in many other countries.

THE PUBLIC AND REPRODUCTIVE POLICY

The apparent inability or unwillingness of the existing political institutions to deal with the issues of reproduction underscores the broader concern that the democratic process is incapable of achieving democratic control over the "crucially important and inordinately complex issues of modern technological society" (Forbes 1988:229). According to Robert Dahl:

> What problems like these have in common is that they have enormously important consequences for a vast number of people, they seem to require government decisions of some kind, and in order to make wise decisions, decision-makers need specialized knowledge that most citizens do not possess. (1985:3)

Reproductive technologies, particularly sex preselection, genetic testing, and reversible sterilization, do have the potential to affect either personally or indirectly a large proportion of the population and of future generations. Also, for reasons detailed earlier, these issues require government action if they are to be kept within manageable bounds. While policy makers will need some specialized knowledge in order to make wise decisions, as Dahl states, the heavy value content and intimate personal quality of reproductive issues demands inclusion of a broader public in making policy. These issues force a reevaluation of the way we make decisions in our society and return us to the enduring debate over the role of the public in public policy.

In part due to the perceived inadequacy of existing political institutions to deal with the issues derived from science and technology, there has been a resurgence of demands for effective participation of potentially affected groups in making policy. Dorothy Nelkin (1980:484) suggests that demands for public scrutiny are inevitable "given the policy importance of many areas of scientific research and the growing concern in the biological sciences with basic life processes." The heightened sensitivity to the social implications of genetic and reproductive technological development, and the intensifying fear by some that societal decisions are being made without adequate public input, have produced a growing concern over the question of who should control the critical policy decisions which face us.

Despite efforts to expand public involvement in the policy process through public hearings, institutional review boards, and an array of ad hoc mechanisms, "political institutions of popular, democratic control are inadequate to guide the scientific and technological enterprise and mediate its effects" (Rettig 1982:22). Weiner (1982:81) argues that even though public interest in development of reproductive technologies is high, "opportunities for public participation are often ineffective." Despite the highly visible problems raised by these technologies, there has been little public discussion of the potential consequences of basic reproductive research or new technologies, nor has there been significant public debate on desirable priorities for application. Although this absence of attention in part is due to the fragmented and specialized nature of the public, part of it reflects institutional gaps.

If the public is to have a positive role, as many observers of democracy assume, how ought this role best be manifested in decisions about the problems inherent in reproductive technology? Moreover, who should be included in the "public" that establishes policies and controls and how ought these controls be organized and applied? Also, while it is popular to express a desire for aggrandizing the role of the public, is there a risk in putting too much faith in the public's desire or ability to accept this responsibility?

The Public Role in Democratic Theory

According to classical democratic theory, the health of a democracy depends upon the existence of a politically informed and active citizenry and its capacity to develop informed opinions about policies and to take an active role in putting such policies into effect. Active, informed participation of all citizens was central to the relatively homogeneous Greek city-state; however, as society became larger and more complex, intense forms of participation in policy making became the domain of a limited number of persons. Instead of accepting responsibility for a full share in public life, political participation for most citizens of the United States shifted to less demanding and less frequent involvement, primarily manifested in the vote. Representative democracy necessarily replaced the more direct forms of control of Greece and Rome. Although the classical ideal public is unlikely to exist in an impersonal and heterogeneous population of 240 million persons, the goal of broad public involvement in policies affecting society as a whole remains central to a democratic value system.

Despite considerable disagreement at the policy level, a consensual political culture that reflects the liberal tradition of John Locke as applied by the framers of the Constitution continues to exist in the United States (Devine 1972). The liberal tradition is not the ideology of a single faction, but rather encompasses liberals and conservatives alike. Although public policy varies over time, it continues to be shaped by this liberal value system under which individuals, personally and collectively, exercise a positive role in the policy of government.

Of all the rules within the liberal tradition, "the one that the people should ultimately control policy is most central" (Devine 1972:143). Although conceptions of popular rule vary, popular consent as an ideal is universally accepted under this value tradition. In addition to its importance as a means of governing, popular participation serves a practical educative function and leads to the self-development of each participating citizen. Democratic character is nurtured through participation. Moreover, public confidence in policy decisions is secured through direct and active citizen participation. The framers of the Constitution institutionalized the value of popular rule through representation, and it remains at the heart of our political culture, even though it is seldom attained in specific policy making.

Alternative Democratic Models

In order to fit classical democratic theory to practice in a contemporary society, it is critical to make adjustments. As soon as one moves away from the pure model, however, there exists a range of possibilities that results in disagreement. A major source of controversy centers on to what degree the public as a whole should make public policy. Figure 7.3 presents a continuum of potential power distributions that currently frame the debate over the role of the public. As one moves to the right on the continuum from demo-

FIGURE 7.3. Models of Democracy: A Continuum

Democratic Egalitarianism	Pluralistic Elite	Technocratic Elite	Ruling Class (nondemocratic)
Many		Few	One

cratic egalitarianism toward a ruling class, the distance from the pure democratic model widens and popular control decreases.

Under democratic egalitarianism, all people rule because they are all equal in capacity and interest in politics. Aristotle moderated this by opting for rule by the middle class in a polity. As noted earlier, U.S. political culture has imbued the public with control over government, based on the assumption that, if given the opportunity, each citizen would have the knowledge and capacity to run the government. Intricate linkage mechanisms, including elections and political parties, have been established to provide the public with the means of popular control, on the premise that the people themselves contain the wisdom necessary for making democratic policy. Democracy, here, not only refers to the means of governing but also introduces the notion of the quality of the decisions, by envisioning democracy as a way of life. The underlying assumption of democratic egalitarianism is that even though the people collectively might make mistakes, it is necessary to give them that opportunity.

Although democratic egalitarianism best fits our political values about government, as noted earlier, it does not fit the facts. Citizens are not equal in either the interest or information necessary to make informed, rational decisions on substantive issues. Most citizens exhibit low levels of interest and participation in the political process, with only the voting in presidential elections even approaching a simple majority of the population. A clear linkage between public opinion and public policy exists on a few visible issues, but that link becomes considerably more nebulous on most issues that are less salient and of little interest to the general public. The result, as Robert Dahl states, is that: "an overwhelming proportion of the citizen body has until quite recently totally abdicated its rights to participate in any way in making nuclear decisions even of the most general sort" (1985:15). According to Miller and associates (1980:29), most investigators of public opinion have "drawn the reluctant conclusion that scientific information is indeed complex and that the educational level of the general population prevents many people from truly understanding the scientific issues of the day." Even if people were capable of acquiring an understanding of the issues, they would lack the time to do so. In fact, few persons are able to become fully informed on more than several issues in our specialized world.

The reality of the public has led to several competing models of

democratic choice that assume that the public interest is best protected, not by mass decisions, but rather by policy made by specialized elites who have the knowledge necessary to make informed
decisions. The technocratic elite approach emphasizes the democratic ends rather than the means of making the decision. Technocracy is rule by technically competent professionals. Proponents of
this model argue that a technocratic elite is essential because of
inherent limitations on the capacity of the public to make technical
decisions. The origin of this approach can be traced to Pareto's
(1935) "sum of outstanding talents." For Pareto, democracy is an
organizational impossibility. Instead, decisions must be made by
experts in each area who have the necessary expertise, interest, and
information to make an informed decision in the public interest.
Technocracy is democratic only in that the elite is "open," because
a technical and professional education is generally available. "All"
one has to do to have influence in an area is to obtain the "proper"
education, which is assumed to be accessible. Conversely, it is
restrictive in the sense that education and, normally, some status
in a hierarchical organization are prerequisites to participation.

Walter Lippmann (1945) moderated the concept of technocracy,
in that the technocrat becomes an elite within a specific substantive area but one who is ultimately accountable to the democratic
public. For Lippmann, the public is too uninformed, uninterested,
and slow to react to help make the complex decisions of the twentieth century. Modern problems require a degree of knowledge
beyond the technical capacity of both individuals and their elected
representatives. Although the public is given a "recruiting function," the policy function is reserved for the experts. Despite his
addition of the accountability of the technocrats to a broader public, for Lippmann rational government in a highly technological
age must center on that segment of society which is most informed
—the technocrats.

Another model of democracy, which falls somewhere between
democratic egalitarianism and technocracy on the continuum is
termed pluralism. Although it does not achieve the optimal democratic form, a pluralistic system provides ultimate popular veto
power on actions of government while allowing those citizens with
specialized interests and abilities to initiate policy proposals in
substantive areas. Pluralism is based primarily on an economic
model of humans which assumes that limited time and resources
must be allocated to maximize both monetary and psychological

rewards for individuals. As a result, most people are reluctant to devote the considerable time or resources necessary to become informed at high levels about particular policy issues or politics in general because the issues appear to be of relatively low priority in terms of payoffs for the average person.

Pluralism also assumes that those individuals who are interested and informed in a specific substantive area are able to establish an interest group through which to pursue their objectives and, furthermore, that all groups have access to the policy makers. The democratic theory behind pluralism is that public decision making is based upon the resolution of conflict between contending groups rather than at the individual level. This concept of competition can be traced to Madison's treatment of factions in *The Federalist Papers*, number 10, where he contends that the best way to guard against control by one faction is to ensure the existence of many competing factions. Theoretically, this clash of special interests ultimately will protect the public interest, although in reality such results seem unlikely. Lowi (1969) and others attack pluralism on this ground, arguing that it serves the interests of the powerful special interests which generally monopolize policy making in each narrow area. Instead of benefiting the public interest, pluralism results in dominance of the policy process by narrow specialized interests at the expense of the public.

Despite the emphasis on interest groups in U.S. society, effective participation in them is limited to that small proportion of the population with sufficient motivation, skills, and time. Even among those with strong feelings on an issue, few are able to influence a group directly. Moreover, access to the decision makers is not as open as the proponents of pluralism contend. Those groups that are able to expend resources consistently over a period of years gain inordinate influence over specific issue areas, while other groups are largely excluded from exerting influence.

In order to refine the description of interest groups, Best (1973:176ff) makes a distinction between stable, multi-interest groups that seek to influence policy over a long period of time, and single-issue groups created and dissolved with great rapidity in their quest to influence a specific decision. According to Best, ad hoc, single-issue groups are the most effective vehicles for expression of public opinion because they arise out of concern for one issue and focus on a narrowly defined political objective upon which the membership agrees. Their ability to mobilize and reflect public opinion, however, is not often translated into actual influence over policy decisions because these groups generally experience difficulty in gaining access to decision makers and in establishing legitimacy and building resources. In order to gain access, the single-issue group must expand its appeal and increase its membership. Ironically, in the process of becoming a multi-interest group, it loses its ability to serve as a vehicle for public opinion. As it becomes involved in a broader range of issues and expands its base, the division of labor within the group becomes institutionalized. Leaders become most interested in perpetuating themselves in power to achieve their own political goals. At the same time, they attempt to satisfy the membership by providing it with primarily nonpolitical benefits and to maintain control of the internal lines of communication.

As a result of this process, lobbying activities of the large, influential organizations seldom represent an articulation of the interests of the group membership, much less the public interest. Instead, they reflect the interests of the leadership, which might or might not be identical to those of the members. Despite the appearance and claims that interest groups protect "the public interest" or even "a public's interest," often the most politically successful groups fall far short of that pluralistic ideal.

The Attentive Public

Although there are still many proponents of democratic egalitarianism, policy is most often made within a framework which more closely approximates one of the two elite models. The nature of the public in these models takes on a form unlike that found in traditional democratic theory. According to Almond (1960:139) the "attentive public" is the relevant democratic public for U.S. society. Instead of having one public which is politically interested and informed, we have many publics with varying degrees of attention to particular issues. The attentive public for Almond is that segment of the public that is informed and interested in political issues in general. Members of the attentive public talk about politics, engage in political activities, have a general interest in politics, and are relatively well-informed about political issues. Within this public, more specialized attentive publics are composed of people attuned to specific issue areas who normally act through groups. In other words, there is a hierarchy of attentiveness or interest even within the general attentive public.

Although Devine (1970:30) admits that theoretically the size of the attentive public is "inexhaustibly expandable to the limits of the population," in practice, at most a quarter of the population can be counted in its ranks, depending on the way attentiveness is measured. Key (1961:546) notes the relevance of this stratum of the attentive because "obviously the highly attentive publics, as they monitor the actions of government and let their judgments be known, play a critical role in assuring a degree of responsiveness of government to nongovernmental opinion." Similarly, Devine (1970) found that policy reflects most closely the views of those who have information, hold opinions, and at least occasionally communicate with the government. Although this is not at all surprising, it does signify major implications for the application of democracy to reproductive policy making in the United States. There exists a division of labor in interest and awareness that severely limits the number of persons who are able to exert any influence over public policy. The low importance of political issues to the mass public necessitates directing efforts to increase public involvement toward more select attentive publics and, at the same time, trying to expand the size of the attentive public. Almond (1960) concludes that since it is impossible for all citizens to be actively involved in all policy areas, specialized publics are essential. However, the general public must retain a "final veto authority," should it be motivated to apply it.

Miller et al. (1980:291) estimate the attentive public for science and technology policy in general is approximately 20 percent of the population. However, that should be seen as an outside figure, because the size of the attentive public on a specific issue depends on how the issue is presented by the government. Although attentiveness is a self-selected attribute, the way in which an issue is framed can influence the scope of participation both in quantity and intensity. If the issues are kept technical and the policy making structure routine, the saliency of the issues will remain subdued and the attentive public small. Also, Miller et al. (1980:292) feel that although access to the attentive publics of science and technology for interested citizens presently is high, institutional mechanisms should be used to maximize recruitment to the ranks of the attentive.

The Role of the Public in Reproductive Policy Making

There is an urgent need for conceptual clarification of the applicability of public control for the separate dimensions of reproductive technology policy making. To do this requires a clear distinction between making technical decisions requiring substantial expertise and establishing broad social priorities. The first depends on technical competence; the second depends on moral competence. Figure 7.4 combines this specialized-generalized continuum with the models of democracy to help us arrive at a meaningful conceptual starting point for analyzing the role of the public in reproductive policy making.

Given the technical complexity of new technologies in human genetics and reproduction, it is highly unlikely that more than a small proportion of the public has the capacity or the inclination to acquire the expertise needed to make decisions concerning research and development of the techniques or regulation of their use. It is critical to remember, however, that new developments in reproduction represent a social as well as a technological revolution. Their potential impact on social values and structures—on the very way we think about individuals and society—is limitless. As noted by Lappé and Martin (1978), science is a "social enterprise" with broad moral and social consequences. As I have argued, we cannot look at any single technology apart from the social and political context within which it is applied. A major component of the issues surrounding reproductive technology, therefore, centers on the broad social dimension on the right end of the continuum in figure 7.4.

The weakest case for egalitarian democracy is in quadrant I. Continued low levels of scientific and technological literacy exhibited by the populace (Miller 1989) make it questionable that many citizens are able or willing to develop a familiarity with the technical aspects of reproductive technology. Only when they become potential users is there the likelihood of them to be drawn into the attentive public. Furthermore, it is likely that the size of the attentive public on the highly technical aspects will be severely constrained. Although social egalitarians argue that active public participation is essential in all aspects of policy making, their effort would better be directed toward influencing the broader decisions of setting social priorities which, in turn, will shape future applications.

FIGURE 7.4. Public Role in Making Policy

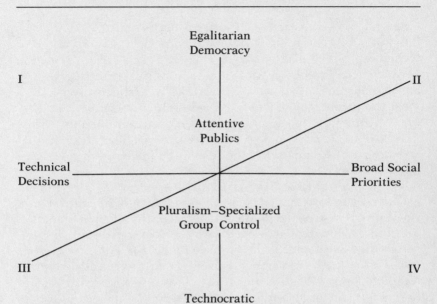

Similarly, technocrats have no valid claim to monopolize decision making in quadrants II and IV, which is dependent on moral —not technical—competence. Expertise in a technical area does not ensure, and in some cases might even obscure, attentiveness to the social implications of technology. The kind of specialized knowledge experts have is not adequate in itself to deal with the unique ethical value dimensions of these issues. For public policy makers to defer to the experts on these decisions courts disaster. While technical experts must be included in the debate over social priorities, and, in fact, might take the lead in a public debate, extensive public involvement is most critical here—the closer we approach full participation, the better for democracy.

Realistically then, quadrants II and III represent the focus in the debate over public participation. The 45 degree line through these quadrants represents the optimal levels of public involvement in reproductive policy. Although the size and quality of the attentive public should be widened at all levels, as we move from the establishment of binding social priorities toward making highly technical decisions, more and more specialized groups take on greater importance. As we shift from deciding what the right ends of social policy ought to be to how to carry out these goals, the scope of participation, by necessity, narrows. Even here, however, policy makers must assure inclusion of all concerned groups, especially representing the interests of persons who are most vulnerable to potential abuse.

Public Control: The Continuing Debate

Although demands for greater public participation and control of technological policy appear to have considerable momentum at present, not all observers are enamored of this trend. Donald Frederickson (1978:80), former director of the National Institutes of Health, cautions against the "dangerous illusion" of a total faith in public control of technology and contends that there are critical limits to "public governance of science." Another danger of making the decision process "too" participatory is that inordinate attention might be given to well-organized interests or to those groups able to gain the attention of public officials and convince them that they speak for the public. According to Lowrance (1982:116):

> To oppose closed bureaucratic procedures is usually legitimate, but it is a lot harder to devise proceedings that are not only open to the affected polity but that encourage extensive "public" participation without just opening channels for special-interest lobbying.

Other critics view these current attempts to expand public control with skepticism and as a means for delaying or blocking technological applications, rather than as objective evaluative mechanisms. They fear cooptation by groups opposed to specific applications. Especially in times of rapid inflation and high interest rates, the advantage of broad public participation might be offset by the high costs imposed by delays when large investments are involved. According to the Organization for Economic Cooperation and Development (1981:97), "inflation has placed a powerful new weapon in the hands of intervenors against the development of large scale technologies."

As a result, many observers emphasize self-governance by experts, an approach corresponding closely to the technocratic elite model. For instance, Price (1978) favors maintenance of the present system of peer review rather than drastic moves toward wider public involvement in specific technological decisions. The assumption is that only experts have the knowledge essential to make the complex technical decisions required today and, thus, they bear the responsibility for making policy. Others go further and argue that scientists have a guaranteed freedom of inquiry implied in the U.S. Constitution or that experts have a contract of sorts with the public through which citizens willingly delegate to experts their democratic right to control science and in turn receive the benefits accrued from technology. Ira Carmen (1986), for example, contends that the public does not have, either directly or through its elected representatives, a right to limit the enterprise of biotechnology even when public funds are involved. Although this logic might be attractive to supporters of a technocratic model, there is no clear foundation for this contract language in the liberal tradition.

Public Control and Reproductive Technologies: Conclusions

The debate over who should control reproductive technology policy will persist within the context of the public's role in science and technology in general. It is meaningful to examine this controversy as a conflict between two democratic models, both of which fall short of the democratic egalitarian ideal. On the one hand are supporters of a technocratic elite model, which reserves to experts the responsibility of making technical decisions. Experts alone, it is argued, have the interest and knowledge necessary to make informed decisions on these difficult and complicated problems. To expand public control is to invite trouble, because the public is uninformed, uninterested, and, therefore, ignorant on these matters.

To contrast, proponents of broadened public control contend that the public is as qualified as the experts to make policy decisions on issues that are as much social and moral as they are technical. The extensive social consequences of specific technological applications warrant close public scrutiny. Although there is a tendency for some supporters of public control to assume that the entire public ought to be involved in policy making, given our understanding of "the public," it is more reasonable to define the public as composed of more or less specialized "attentive" publics. A pluralistic-type elite model, therefore, seems to be a more meaningful alternative than democratic egalitarianism to the technocratic elite option espoused by those opposed to broadened public involvement.

Although one can speak of expanding the potential attentive public on a particular issue by framing it in readily understandable terms and educating the public to the potential options and the consequences of each, it is unrealistic and probably a waste of valuable effort to attempt to integrate the entire mass public into the policy-making process in any direct manner. Energies, instead, should be directed toward ensuring that every person who is attentive to a specific issue area has the opportunity to participate meaningfully. The task, then, is to provide public mechanisms through which interested members of the public can become informed and, at the same time, enjoy more than a token role in formulating policy choices. Although it is not practical to approach the degree of public awareness and participation necessary for the democratic egalitarian model, it is possible—given our knowledge of the public attentive to science and technology—to expand the base of interest and control substantially. This can be accomplished by altering existing public decision-making institutions so that they are more open and responsive to public demands and by designing new mechanisms to maximize public input.

Before any mechanism can maximize public involvement in technologically oriented decisions, there is a need for more effective means of educating the public. The technical nature of many of the issues in reproduction are beyond the expertise of those not trained in the specific field. However, if framed with care, even these issues can be understood by a relatively broad attentive public. Weiner (1982:90) sees the experts themselves as crucial initiators of public discussion. Because of their knowledge, experts can identify at an early stage possible problems related to their work— even if in the short run this makes it more difficult—and participate with other groups to make choices consistent with more inclusive public value systems.

One problem in educating the public on the technical aspects of the issues is the presence of glaring differences of opinion regarding scientific facts among the experts themselves. Rettig (1982:23) sees this lack of elite consensus on "the appropriate response to a number of key policy issues affecting the scientific and technological enterprise" as a critical shortcoming since "without such consensus, clear signals cannot be given . . . and popular support for agreed-upon policies cannot be generated." In each policy area, there are cases where lack of agreement on scientific facts that are relevant to public and official understanding of the issue fuels debate over use of the technology. Because existing institutions are dependent on some form of expert testimony, when the experts disagree, confusion results. Moreover, since those who testify often represent groups that have an obvious stake in the policy decision, it is not surprising that they interpret scientific fact in a way that is favorable to their position. The escalating claims of expert opponents often appear to generate enormous uncertainty in the minds of the public.

Ironically, one unintended consequence of efforts to inform the public about reproductive issues might be to increase demand for such services. A well-educated public might well be one that places considerably more pressure on the government to guarantee access to technologies, even though in so doing they jeopardize the interests of future generations. The quest for perfect children as part of a search for "happiness through the endless gratification of desire, particularly through the acquisition and consumption of things" (Dahl 1985:27) could work counter to the goals of those persons urging more public involvement. Instead of resulting in a more balanced, thoughtful policy of reproduction, this course could trigger an entrepreneurial response that makes regulation even more difficult as providers rush to fill the growing demand.

CHAPTER EIGHT

Toward a Rational
Reproductive Policy

THE FOREGOING discussion of the issues surrounding the dramatic progression of developments in human genetic and reproductive technology illustrates the scope of their impact on the future. In spite of the benefits they offer many people, however, numerous applications threaten to undermine traditional values, thus generating opposition from many quarters. This combination of a growing demand for reproductive technologies on the one hand, and adamant condemnation on the other, guarantees that the issues enumerated here will not dissipate.

More than any other area of technology in the 1990s, human reproduction innovations force us to reevaluate prevailing assumptions that are no longer appropriate. Moreover, they require serious considerations for making changes in the policy structure to allow flexible responses to even more resounding developments of the future. These technologies also challenge traditional notions of individual rights and raise concerns about commercialization of the very essence of human life, procreation. In addition to the need to clarify social priorities and raise the public consciousness about these new issues, public mechanisms must be established to assess and monitor these technological advances on a continuing, instead of the current, ad hoc, basis. Similarly, it is essential that potential benefits and risks associated with each technique be defined and evaluated as soon as feasible in the developmental process, before they become widely diffused.

It is by no means too early to set social priorities regarding reproductive research and application. In vitro fertilization, surrogate motherhood, sex preselection, long-term contraceptive implants, and an array of other reproductive intervention applications soon will be available to those persons who desire them, and perhaps applied to those persons who do not. Moreover, the use of prenatal diagnostic and genetic screening techniques is expanding rapidly, as are fetal therapy and surgery. The not-so-remote future promises evermore sophisticated means of intervening in human reproduction. Without clear notions of desired social priorities and long-term goals, attempts to guide or channel these innovations will be futile. The response to these new policy problems must be decisive but creative because, without such action, the reproductive revolution promises to get quickly out of control.

This chapter explains what steps should be undertaken to deal with the challenges of new reproductive intervention capabilities. We must learn to sharpen societal goals for the future. What do we want from society and what are we willing to sacrifice or pay to attain those goals? In chapter 1, I argued that, given the trends in technology, we can proceed either toward a brave new world or to a world of greater individual choice. The direction we take is dependent more on political and social decisions than on technological advances.

Unfortunately, at present we seem to want it all—we want the advantages that technologies promise to fix our problems, but we are largely unwilling to set clear boundaries as to where these technologies are taking us. Put another way, we are too willing to let technologies shape our future rather than our directing the course of technological development. Society, therefore, is not in control of the very powers that are shaping our destiny.

Furthermore, the pluralist approach to political decision making narrows our vision to the near time and space and needlessly drains our capacity to be as creative and innovative in the political sphere as we are in the technological sphere. The political institutions, which may have served us well in simpler times are not sufficient to handle the complex problems of a rapidly changing world. This should not be taken as an indictment solely of the U.S. political system because all nations are having similar difficulties with reproductive technologies. As discussed in chapter 6, however, parliamentary systems seem in general to be structurally better fitted to deal with these politically explosive problems. In any case, we must be open to effecting changes in the way we make policy decisions, even to the extent of modifying existing institutions, should that be necessary.

SHAPING FUTURE TECHNOLOGY DIRECTIONS

It is important to understand that we can, indeed, shape the boundaries and future directions of human genetic and reproductive technologies. There is a tendency upon examining the rapidity and scope of technological change to assume that its very momentum is so powerful that it denies society the capacity to manage and direct its development. Although history shows that the ability to control technology is difficult and that despair is understandable, if society so desires, significant control is possible.

One theme of this book is that the revolution in reproductive technologies is altering our values concerning children, the family, and the meaning of human life itself. While it is true that technologies transform values and the way we think about things, the relationship between values and technology is reciprocal—values also shape the boundaries of technology. For example, SM became an issue in the 1980s, not because of some dramatic breakthrough in technology, but rather because of an underlying change in the way we think about reproduction. The technique for effectuating SM as largely practiced today, AID, has been in existence for over a century, but surrogacy contracts became common only in the last decade after childless couples found adoption difficult. Also contributing to the demand of SM and other applications was a re-emergence in the last decade of the importance of genetic roots and the attainment of sufficient wealth by young professionals to afford these expensive fertility interventions. There is also evidence (Lor-

ber 1987) that technically IVF could have come considerably earlier than 1978. Human eggs were actually fertilized ex utero as
early as the 1940s, but research was phased out because of a hostile
social climate. Deeper value changes that can be speculated to have
set the stage for TMRs relate to the "me-centered" values of the
baby boom generation that demand gratification of desires through
technology.

Likewise, the acceptance of, or demand for, a wide range of
prenatal diagnosis, genetic screening, and reproductive-mediating
technologies is heightened by the trend toward one- or two-chil-
dren families. While the "perfect child" mentality discussed earlier
has been encouraged by advances in technology, it has also been a
powerful force behind the diffusion of the technologies. This quest
for the perfect child can be traced to smaller families which, in
turn, reflect the changing image of the family brought on by the
economic realities of raising children, a concern for population
control, and drastically altered lifestyles.

Technologies, then, might take on a life of their own, but only if
the social climate is agreeable. If it can be argued that the 1960s
was ripe for the contraceptive revolution, it is clear that in the
1980s society was open to the second reproductive revolution described in this book. The initial and almost unbridled enthusiasm
for these new intervention capabilities has given way in many
quarters to a sober realization that these remarkable technologies
bring with them problems as well as benefits.

It is important to remember, however, that in all vital areas we
humans exercise considerable effort to serve our own good by exerting control over nature. If, as some observers (Hartigan 1987)
contend, procreation is the most important reason for human existence and societies are organized primarily to facilitate that purpose, then reproduction is an area of direct relevance to the continued survival of society. There is no defense for leaving fertility or
infertility up to chance when both overpopulation and childlessness bring misery. In fact, it can be argued that if we have the
means to intervene and thus ameliorate natural problems but fail
to use them, we surrender to those very forces that we strive to
overcome in all other areas of life. The move from chance to purpose in reproduction is unavoidable within the long tradition of
human desire to control nature through technology. The burden of
proof, therefore, is on those persons who question where this is all
leading us.

REGULATING REPRODUCTIVE TECHNOLOGIES

Despite the critical problems reproductive interventions raise for society and the difficult policy issues they create, it is both undesirable and unlikely that they be prohibited. First, a prohibition of the use of any single application would be problematic within a constitutional framework that places heavy emphasis on procreative freedom. Second, banning use of a technique in one jurisdiction, whether state or county, is unlikely to deter its use in other jurisdictions. The major impact of prohibiting a particular application would be to further the gap between those who have the funds to go elsewhere and those who do not. Third, prohibiting the use of a technology out of concern for its undesired consequences could foreclose the possibility of beneficial consequences in other applications.

While prohibition of individual use of available techniques is unfeasible, and perhaps counterproductive, concern over misuse of a technique or over the negative long-term aggregate consequences should result in strict regulatory efforts, coupled with comprehensive education efforts, to channel these technologies into socially acceptable uses. To some extent we have over the last decade made strides in this direction regarding reproductive control technologies, especially sterilization. Although there remain instances of abuse of involuntary sterilization, by providing administrative mechanisms to protect those persons or groups most vulnerable to exploitation, sterilization for most persons represents an expansion of individual choice. Prohibiting the use of sterilization techniques would be undesirable even if it was feasible. New developments in technology, such as long-term subdermal implants, however, require continuous attention to potential abuse as do other human genetic and reproductive innovations.

The major policy problem with TMRs is to create public mechanisms to protect the interests of all parties, especially those most vulnerable to exploitation and abuse. Present use patterns of these technologies raise concerns of class discrimination. Feminists, minority group leaders, and civil libertarians have legitimate fears concerning the way in which these technologies are applied. Clearly, there is a danger that while reproductive technologies expand the procreative choices of affluent middle-class (largely white) couples who use them with free informed consent, they threaten those same freedoms of the less affluent who have access to them only within a context of social control. In particular, poor women who are dependent on the state for financial support are vulnerable.

This potential for abuse requires careful monitoring of the circumstances under which technologies are employed across socioeconomic and racial lines and considerably more public commitment to be intolerant of misuse. Although our system has in many ways been well served by the free market system, commercialization of reproductive services threatens to exacerbate social inequities and undermine efforts to adequately regulate these technologies. Again, however, the answer is not to ban the use of the techniques but rather to ensure that proper standards are enforced to protect all parties.

We must look carefully at the relationship of those seeking and those providing reproductive services. Consumers must be protected against exploitation. In the health care arena, this is largely accomplished through professional associations and state licensing. The right to practice medicine is contingent on compliance with standards set by medical societies and licensing authorities. Although TMRs are presented as medical interventions, however, in part because of their newness, adequate state control has not been established.

Furthermore, while the professional guidelines established by AFS, AATB, and ACOG are valuable controls over those providers who choose to affiliate with them, they are in no way binding on all enterprises offering the technologies. Part of the reason for this is that many of the most used TMRs are not medical procedures. As noted earlier, self-administered AID or administration of it by lay persons is practiced. Also, SM is a legal construction, not a medical one. What this means is that these applications can be made outside the medical establishment. The fact that many continue to be made within that realm attests to the symbolic significance of medicalization, not technical realities.

REPRODUCTIVE TECHNOLOGIES AND FUTURE GENERATIONS

The problem of shifting conceptions of parental responsibility becomes even more complicated when the effects of parents' present actions on descendants beyond their immediate offspring are considered. Deciding whether to engineer a profound change in an expected or newborn child is difficult enough; if the change is inheritable, the burden of responsibility could be truly awesome.

The above quotation from the final report on genetic engineering of the President's Commission for the Study on Ethical Problems in Medicine and Biomedical and Behavioral Research (1982:65) cogently frames the issue of what responsibility present generations have for the well-being of future generations. Moreover, as the technological capacities to control the products of procreation grow, assumptions of what constitutes a normal functioning human on the one hand, and what counts as a serious defect or disability on the other, will result in further changes in the concept of what society owes to children and future generations.

In light of all the difficulties in balancing the rights and obligations of those now living and the preoccupation of political institutions with the present and near future, it should not be surprising that concern for the remote future is inhibited. Until now, the answer to the above question as reflected in reproductive policy is that concern for future generations, even for the direct product, the children, plays a minor role at best in setting contemporary social priorities. Brewer and deLeon see this as a mistake because all policy is future oriented. "Human beings continually orient themselves to the future, and policy is one manifestation . . . of the collective perception of the future" (Brewer and deLeon 1983:107). Therefore, determination of who the relevant participants in the policy process are may involve many who do not yet exist. Although addition of the future dimension to current policy making incurs some costs in complexity, "that reason alone should not obscure the point that current policy decisions have significant consequences for future generations which must be taken into account today" (Brewer and deLeon 1983:17).

There continues to be disagreement over the extent to which obligations toward future generations ought to influence contemporary societal policy. Kieffer (1975:86) argues that, at a minimum, the living have an obligation to refrain from any action that endangers future generations' enjoyment of the same rights now assumed. Proper moral concern is not limited to the near neighbor, but also the distant neighbor in space and time. We must be aware of any processes that might be irreversibly harmful for future human life. In like manner, Feinberg (1974) contends that we have a strong obligation to posterity out of respect for their rights as humans. In his view, we do not have a right to deprive future generations of the necessary conditions for life as we know it, even if this requires restrictions on certain freedoms of those now living.

The opposing position is that primary obligation is to more immediate generations and not to hypothetical populations. Just as the present generation has had to adapt to the effects of decisions made in the past, so future generations must adapt to decisions made now. Most adherents of this viewpoint agree that no decisions should be made that intentionally endanger the rights and survival of future humans, but it is often argued that first concern must be for persons now living and their immediate offspring. This posture encourages only minimal restraints upon actions based solely on the fate of those in the distant future. For Golding (1968:457),

> It is highly doubtful that we have an obligation to establish social programs that would secure a "good life" (prevent the undesirable, promote the desirable) for the community of the "remote" future. The conditions of life then are likely to be so different from any that we can now imagine that we do not know what to desire for them.

As a result, conflicts between the promotion of the good of nearby generations and of remote generations should be resolved in favor of the former.

This second viewpoint is less tenable under current conditions because today's actions have impressive potential to constrain or broaden the alternatives open in the future. Decisions made in the near future will unalterably limit or expand the decisions of all those who follow. Moreover, the irreversibility of reproductive intervention makes the necessity for consideration of future generations even more crucial. According to Gustafson (1974:213), advances in knowledge of human genetics and the ability to intervene is magnifying this responsibility. He argues that "present generations are 'causally' responsible to some extent for the genetic health of future generations, and thus it can be argued that they also have a 'moral' responsibility to them."

An Ethics of Responsibility to the Future

The revolution brought on by the new capacity to intervene in human genetics and reproduction also challenges the very bases of western ethics. Traditional ethics assumed that human nature remained more or less constant. It also presupposed that the sphere of human action did not reach beyond the present and immediate. As stated by Hans Jonas,

> All enjoinders and maxims of traditional ethics, materially different as they may be, show this confinement to the immediate setting of action. . . . The ethical universe is composed of contemporaries and its horizon to the future is confined by the foreseeable span of their lives. (1984:5)

Under these ethical frameworks, no one was held responsible for the unintended future effects of his or her well-intentioned acts. The timespan of foresight, goal setting, and accountability was short, and proper conduct was defined by immediate or near consequences only. The long-run of consequences beyond was left to chance or fate, not human action.

In the wake of modern technology, however, all of this has drastically and irreparably changed. For Jonas (1984:6), "modern technology has introduced actions of such novel scale, objects, and consequences that the framework of former ethics can no longer contain them." With the new-found powers we have to reshape nature, disrupt the ecological balance, and alter the human condition comes the corresponding ethical responsibility for the exercise of these powers. Reproductive technology is at the center of this dramatic expansion of the range of human action and, thus, the new responsibility toward future generations.

In response to modern technology, Jonas sets forth a theory of responsibility for both the private and public sphere. The axiom is that "responsibility is a correlate of power and must be commensurate with the latter's scope and that of its exercise" (1984:x). Moreover, the discharge of this responsibility requires lengthened foresight, a "scientific futurology." The irreversible and cumulative character of technological intervention, unrecognized in traditional ethics, mandates an extension of the relevant horizon of responsibility to the indefinite future where the impact of these interventions is likely to be most felt. Past technologies have shown the vulnerability of nature to human intervention, but often only after damage has already been done. The long-term implications of genetic intervention, especially, demand knowledge commensurate with the causal scale of action. Although there is no complete knowledge of the future upon which to base our decisions, neither is there complete ignorance. In any case, we can not opt out of our responsibility to the future by claiming ignorance.

This new ethics of responsibility also entails supplanting the traditional concept of reciprocal duty with that of nonreciprocity of duties. Conventional ideas of rights and duties, which assume that those who do not yet exist cannot make claims upon those persons who do, no longer hold in light of the powers we have to constrain the options of all posterity. Although reciprocity is the hallmark of traditional rights and duties, Jonas (1984:39) contends that the "archetype of all responsible action," powerfully implanted in us by nature, is the nonreciprocal duty of parent to child. Although parents might expect reciprocity after the child reaches adulthood, it is not a precondition or motive for their responsibility owed the child. Just as parental responsibility is a one-way relationship to dependent progeny, so political responsibility of the present is a one-way relationship to the future, not the mutual relationship between independent adults. Unlike parental responsibility, under which childrearing has a definite substantive goal terminating in the independence of the adult child, however, political responsibility has no point of termination. No intrinsic terminus is set for political responsibility, or for mankind as a whole, by the nature of its object, because there is no such predetermined goal as in parenthood (Jonas 1984:108).

Under the ethics of responsibility, unlike previous ethics, an agent's concrete moral responsibility at the time of action extends far beyond its proximate effects. How far it extends, for Jonas (1984:107), depends upon the nature of the object and on the extent of our power and prescience. As our capacity to intervene directly in the human genome expands and our power over future generations heightens, the time span of our responsibility widens appreciably. "In fact, the changed nature of human action changes the very nature of politics" (Jonas 1984:9).

Reproductive Policy Making and the Future

Especially in regard to reproductive intervention techniques, responsibility to future generations must become an integral aspect of any policy. The decisions made in the coming decades are likely not only to modify our conceptions of humanhood, but also to alter the characteristics of future individuals and the prospects of continued survival of the human race. Society can ill afford either to blindly ignore the opportunities presented by reproductive technologies or to actively pursue human reproductive intervention without including futuristic considerations. Many of the recipients of the benefits of today's research are tomorrow's citizens. Unfortunately, potential harmful effects of such research might irreversibly affect those same generations. Policy decisions made now, therefore, must consider, to the maximum extent possible, such concerns. Although it is impractical to make decisions based solely on concepts of obligation to future generations, the awareness that each innovation has broad ramifications on future alternatives ought to raise our consciousness regarding that goal. In the words of Wenk:

> People are part of the decision apparatus. Unless they are willing to trade off instant gratification for some vision of future benefits for humankind generally, and for their own progeny specifically, we will indeed be in difficulty. Unless the public embeds the future in its decision calculus, the political leadership will remain in the vise of the short run. The hazard then exists of action or inaction which could debase individual integrity or extinguish humanity altogether. Even before that may happen, the benign neglect of the future may undermine even the future capacity to decide. (1981:269)

The integration of a proper concern for the future into the policy-making process necessitates substantial alterations in the way we as a society make decisions. In fact, this new responsibility casts doubt on the capacity of representative government, as now practiced, to meet these demands (Jonas 1984:22). Under a pluralist system, only present interests make themselves heard and felt and require consideration. Especially on issues as complex and emotionally charged as reproduction, single-issue interest groups become active, vocal, and influential. With few exceptions, their concern is with the near term or immediate, not the distant, future. Also, because public officials are held accountable to their constituencies of the present, future-oriented policy gives way to placating those persons and groups whose demands are loudest. Because the interests of the day hold sway, the future is nowhere represented.

The concerns raised by human genetic and reproductive intervention demand attention to long-range and remote interests of the as yet nonexistent future members of humanity. However,

The nonexistent has no lobby, and the unborn are powerless. Thus accountability to them has no political reality behind it in present decision making, and when they can make their complaint, then we, the culprits, will no longer be there. (Jonas 1984:22)

The critical question is what force can represent the future in present policy making? How can we adequately address future interests in a system that is designed to be present-oriented? Practically, what political mechanisms are necessary to lengthen the time frame of policy making in the U.S.?

In order to build a capacity for long-range future planning into the policy process and give us the ability to think systematically about the future, Lester Milbrath (1986) recommends the creation of a special governmental unit designed to provide society with a better understanding of where it is headed and what steps must be taken to get where we want to go. To this end, Milbrath proposes establishing, as part of the national government, a Council for Long-Range Societal Guidance. The special charge of the council would be to look to the long-range consequences of proposed government actions and provide guidance to leaders and citizens. The council would engage in long-range forecasting and develop possible future scenarios. It would also monitor conditions and changes in society, facilitate social learning, enhance citizen dialogue and thinking about the issues, and make recommendations to public officials based on thorough research and deep thought. Milbrath conceives of the council as composed of thirty generalists who have demonstrated a high capacity for thinking about broad social issues. These generalists, however, would be aided by two or more competing forecasting teams and adequate staffing to ensure an open flow of information and ideas. As a result of the council's efforts, the public interest would be "given a greater chance to become defined by careful, intellectual, holistic, long-term analysis, instead of simplistic, sloganized appeals to short-term interests" (Milbrath 1986:24).

Although the specifics of Milbrath's proposal might or might not be feasible or desirable, the concept of a new governmental mechanism to provide a future-oriented dialogue over reproductive issues is attractive. As long as the existing institutions fail to give adequate attention to the initiation and estimation stages of the policy process and are unable or unwilling even to set reasonable priorities and goals for society, resolution of these problems is impossible. I agree strongly with Milbrath that "well-deliberated long-range policies offer better solutions than hasty patchwork actions" (1986:33). Unfortunately, as noted throughout this book, fragmented, piecemeal, and simplistic attempts to deal with the complex problems concerning the reproductive technologies are the norm. The resulting policies continue to fall far short of what is needed as we grapple with continually more difficult decisions.

TECHNOLOGY ASSESSMENT AND FORECASTING

Short of creating a new branch or agency of long-range planning is the interim measure of strengthening our current efforts of technology assessment and forecasting of reproductive technology. Although the need for comprehensive assessment of technological advances has long been recognized, only recently has there been an effort to integrate such considerations into policy making. In spite of establishment of the Office of Technology Assessment by Congress, it is questionable how much influence these assessments have on actual policy.

Technology assessment has been defined, alternately, as a narrow technical analysis that elaborates the technical risks and benefits inherent in a specific technique or an inclusive broad assessment that details the interplay of the technology, social values, and social institutions. Although technical assessments are essential for evaluating options for the application of each reproductive technique, adequate estimation must include the social, moral, and policy dimensions. Because of the interactive and complex nature of reproductive issues, inclusive assessment procedures and mechanisms designed to analyze the nontechnical, as well as technical, effects of a technology are essential.

Coates (1971:225) defines technology assessment as "the systematic study of the effects on society that may occur when a technology is introduced, extended, or modified, with special emphasis on the impacts that are unintended, indirect, and delayed." This definition contains reference to two aspects that are crucial to effective assessment. Most obvious is the broad scope of concern for effects on "society." Second, and more subtle, is the emphasis on second-order consequences: those which are "unintended, indirect, or delayed."

Although there is no single accepted procedure for performing technology assessment, Jones (1971:26) offers a useful seven-step model that includes these components:

1. Defining the assessment task
2. Describing relevant technologies
3. Developing state-of-society assumptions
4. Identifying impact areas
5. Preparing a preliminary impact analysis
6. Identifying possible action options
7. Completing the impact analysis

Step one entails detailing the scope of the inquiry by setting the boundaries as to specific time period, type of impact, and inclusiveness. Step two describes the current state of the technology to be assessed, surveys related technologies, and attempts to estimate the future state of the art and the scope of its use. Step three identifies major nontechnological factors that might influence the development and application of the technologies, while the fourth stage defines the social characteristics that will be most influenced by introduction and use of the technology. Basically, the first four steps establish a framework for the analysis.

The last three steps of technology assessment involve analysis of the anticipated social consequences of the technology. In step five, the analyst posits what social groups and institutions will be affected by the technology and how. Stage six clarifies the alternative courses of action. Attempts are made to develop options that will provide maximum public benefit while reducing to a minimum the negative consequences of the technology being assessed. Finally, in step seven, each option is analyzed as to its social impact, given the potential modifications of this impact by changes outlined in the proceeding step. This process is difficult to accomplish, but it results in an elaboration of the many technical and nontechnical considerations that ought to be, but seldom are, part of each policy decision regarding the development and/or application of a technology.

Much controversy continues to surround technology assessment. One criticism centers on the tendency of conventional assessments to force complex, highly disparate problems into a single predetermined analytical process. In the assessment of four relatively straightforward biomedical technologies, the National Academy of Science (1975:4) concluded: "The breadth and complexity of the subject matter posed serious obstacles to developing a uniform mode of analysis . . . different technologies presented different kinds of problems for analysis and assessment." Moreover, Tribe (1973:627) contends that by emphasizing impacts and outcomes, technology assessment minimizes the role of "soft" variables that cannot be measured easily. As a result, "entire problems tend to be reduced to terms that misstate their underlying structure and ignore the 'global' features that give them their total character." Like any other form of applied policy analysis, technology assessment can become a weapon for the "disguised advancement of narrow interests." Simply broadening the range of factors considered by expanding the spectrum of affected interests, including social costs and benefits, and extending the time frame will not resolve the underlying problems of the instrumental mode of analysis where policy decisions are viewed simply as a product of tradeoffs among existing interests and values in the community.

According to Tribe (1973:624), the policy-analytic mode itself is flawed due to its focus on outcomes at the expense of questions of process. Although he does not dismiss technology assessment entirely, he suggests that emphasis should be placed on what the needs and values ought to be rather than accepting them as givens. If technology assessment and environment analysis cannot address the question of what one's ultimate ends and values ought to be, then they "will either have to be silent as to an increasing significant range of problems that both disciplines should be called upon to illuminate or will mistakenly treat the choice of ultimate ends as though that task were really one calling only for the selection of means to attainment of ends already given" (Tribe 1973:641). According to Ferkiss (1978:4), the difficulties involved with technology assessment are compounded when technology is judged within the context of "political and social goals which are themselves subject to controversy."

In addition to the need to add an explicit constitutive dimension to deal with the critical value problems accompanying all reproductive technologies, there are serious practical constraints. Primary among these limitations are inadequate data, the lack of reliable means of forecasting advances in technology, the inability to determine acceptable risk thresholds, and the inability to predict with accuracy alterations in social values. In spite of the flurry of activity and highly optimistic reports concerning technology assessment, continuing problems center on its ultimate grounding in traditional values, the difficulty of determining the impact of each of a multitude of subtly interrelated variables on society, and the inability to create a socially neutral mechanism for conducting the assessment free from political and social constraints.

A major task in assessing potential social-policy responses to a technological innovation and to the issues its emergence produces is that of reducing uncertainty concerning the long-term consequences of each option. The formulation and analysis of alternative courses of action depend on the ability to predict accurately technological development, as well as to evaluate the impact of each development. Among the means for reducing such uncertainty are a variety of forecasting methods, including time series models and extrapolations, computer simulations, delphi techniques, and scenario-based games. Central to this effort is the inclusion in our decision apparatus of the capacity to forecast what is foreseeable with sophistication and elegance and to contemplate what might be, especially in terms of those futures we wish to avoid. Kass (1981:459) argues that policy makers must "face up to reasonable projections of future accomplishments, consider whether they are cause for social concern, and see whether or not the principles *now* enunciated and the practices *now* established are adequate to deal with any such concerns." Although we can never know with certainty what will happen, much less how soon, uncertainty is not the same as ignorance, because some events seem likely. While prediction is difficult, effort must be taken to analyze the directions in which we are proceeding.

Although it is unlikely that we can make useful proactive reproductive policy without knowledge of future technological developments, there remains considerable disagreement over both the practicality and desirability of technology forecasting. Drucker (1981:251), for example, contends that technology assessment designed to predict remote effects of new technologies is impossible because the "future impact of technology is almost always beyond anybody's imagination." The "dismal record" of social and economic experts, especially in foreseeing technological impact, exists because technology is far more difficult to predict than other developments since its effects result from the convergence of a number of factors only few of which are technological.

Collingridge (1980) agrees that efforts at forecasting the social impact of technologies are wasted because it is not possible to foresee complex interactions between technology and society over a sufficient time span with the certainty necessary to control technology in the present. For Collingridge:

The central research problem concerning the control of technology, is not to find better ways of forecasting the social effects of technology, it is to understand why it is that as technologies develop and become diffused, they become more resistant to controls which seek to alleviate their unwanted social consequences. (1980:23)

POLITICAL FEASIBILITY ANALYSIS

A factor which considerably complicates the task of technology assessment before it can guide policy is the direct political context. As important as reliable estimates of technical feasibility are, more crucial in framing reproductive policy are analyses of the political feasibility of each policy option. According to Webber (1986:545), "While technical soundness of a strategy proposed to solve a controversial policy problem should be a necessary condition for its adoption, policy alternatives that do not have widespread political support are not likely to be adopted."

Valuable resources are wasted in seeking technically feasible solutions without analyzing the political feasibility of each policy option. Therefore, it is critical before pursuing a logically optimal policy to assess the relative likelihood that the policy could actually be adopted and implemented. Moreover, because favorable action is essential at all stages in the policy-making process, political feasibility analysis must examine the relevant actors and events at each stage and anticipate the likely resolution of the policy problem as it moves through the process (Webber 1986:546).

Relevant data in political feasibility efforts include an accurate estimate of what political constraints or support are likely to mobilize in reaction to a particular policy initiative. A proposal is politically feasible if it is acceptable to, or at least not opposed by, a sufficient proportion of the relevant policy makers so that it is likely, although by no means guaranteed, to be adopted. One must weigh which influential groups are likely to support and oppose a proposal. More important than actual numbers is the anticipated intensity of activity. Although anti-abortion groups, for example, represent a small proportion of the population, their often rabid commitment has exaggerated their influence on reproductive policy. Considerably more attention of policy analysts, therefore, must be directed to the political landscape before feasible political activity can be established. Although political feasibility studies are by nature speculative, this is, in fact, one area where significant improvement can be made with minimal expenditure.

The Scope of Political Opposition to Reproductive Interventions

One of the most fascinating political aspects in the public response to reproductive-mediating technologies concerns the configuration of groups skeptical of, or hostile to, these new capacities. Interesting alliances have evolved in opposition to reproductive technologies, alliances traversing traditional liberal-conservative lines. This has resulted in cleavages among traditional political allies and, more importantly, thrust unlikely groups together in their opposition. This pattern has led to considerable uncertainty among policy makers who can no longer count on traditional coalitions for support. They now must deal with an array of single-issue groups that, although having different political agendas, tenuously share a desire to restrict research or application of reproductive and genetic technologies. Figure 8.1 illustrates how this resistance crosses the ideological spectrum. Although not all of the groups composing each category oppose reproductive technologies—and some of those which do, selectively disapprove or approve of particular applications—overall, these groups are, at best, suspicious of the reproductive revolution.

On the right end of the spectrum are those groups which tend to oppose reproductive intervention on moral grounds. They are most clearly represented by right-to-life groups, themselves a unique new coalition of traditionally Democratic Roman Catholics and Republican fundamentalist Protestants. There is no clearer statement of condemnation of these technologies than the March 10, 1987, document of the Vatican's Congregation for the Doctrine of Faith entitled "Instruction on Respect for Human Life in its Origins

---

FIGURE 8.1. An Ideological Continuum of Groups Opposed
to Reproductive Technology

Left	Women's Health Groups	Minority Group Leaders		Religious Leaders	Right to Life Groups	Right
	Civil Libertarians	Handicap Advocacy Groups				

and on the Dignity of Procreation." This reaffirmation of the Vatican's opposition to AI, IVF, SM, embryo freezing, and so forth, is explicit and inflexible. Although there has been vocal dissent from some clergy and widespread disobedience from rank-and-file Catholics, as reflected in their overrepresentation in IVF use, the Church's disapproval has significant policy ramifications.

There is a wide range of views regarding reproductive technologies across Protestant denominations in the United States, with a clear split between the mainline bodies and the more conservative or fundamentalist sects. Less clearly articulated than the official Catholic doctrine, many Protestant leaders and theologians have expressed reservations about the use of technology-mediated reproduction. For instance, some Protestants agree that the use of third-party germ material violates the sanctity of the marriage covenant and that it is tantamount to adultery (van Regenmorter et al., 1986). "Playing God" is a label often applied to reproductive interventions by these religious leaders.

Until now, perhaps because of the attention paid to the abortion issue, these "conservative" groups have been the most salient opponents to reproductive technology. Recently, however, they have been joined by traditionally liberal, or even radical, elements opposed to reproductive intervention out of fear of repression, stigmatization, or invasion of privacy. Minority-group leaders, especially black and Hispanic, as well as some Orthodox Jewish spokespersons, have publicly criticized various genetic and reproductive technologies as counter to the interests of their communities. Black leaders are especially wary of attempts by largely white family planning and health care providers to offer genetic screening and sterilization services to welfare women who are vulnerable to coercive methods. Even abortion is viewed by some black leaders, including presidential candidate Jesse Jackson, as a threat to the black community and as a subtle means of genocide.

Moreover, minority leaders can point to many instances where technologies designed and used by the middle class to expand procreative choice are used to constrain the choices of their members. Their caution and even fear of the reproductive revolution is understandable in light of past policies. For this reason, civil libertarians such as the American Civil Liberties Union have become actively involved in cases dealing with these technologies and have initiated a major research effort on reproductive rights. Likewise, advocacy groups supporting the handicapped, concerned with the impact of reproductive intervention on societal values relating to the quality of life of the handicapped, are becoming mobilized on these issues.

Although feminist groups were late in becoming highly active in the debate over reproductive technologies, in large part because of their preoccupation with abortion, they have become a very salient force of opposition. Their concern over the impact of reproductive technologies on women is natural because in most cases it is women and their children who take the risk. According to Mies (1987:340), reproductive technology

> cannot claim to be neutral; nor is it free from the sexist, racist and ultimately fascist biases in our societies. These biases are built into the technology itself, and they are not merely a matter of its application. Apart from this, an historical continuity of these principles can be traced from the 19th century eugenics movement, to the fascist race politics of the Nazis, to the present day genetic, reproductive and population control technologies.

Although some individual feminists such as Mies are ideologically unalterably opposed to all reproductive technologies as mere extensions of a patriarchal society, most women's organizations focus their criticism toward particular applications or abuses.

As early as 1980, representatives of the National Organization for Women, the National Women's Health Network, and the Federation of Organizations of Professional Women called for a moratorium on the use of in vitro fertilization, sex preselection techniques including those utilizing amniocentesis, and birth-control methods designed only for women (Kotulak, 1980). They noted that women bear increased health risks for these technologies which also threaten women's role in society. Hubbard (1980:12) adds that in vitro fertilization, for instance, is expensive and will "distort our health priorities and funnel scarce resources into a questionable effort." According to Hubbard, "we must find better and less risky solutions for women who want to parent but cannot bear children of their own."

More recently the National Women's Health Network has focused criticism at the commercialization of procreation and the trend toward deterioration of women's procreative rights in the courts. For instance, its board of directors concludes that:

> commercial surrogacy arrangements as contrary to public policy and existing laws, disregard the value of human life, and should be pro-

hibited by law. All surrogacy contracts or agreements should be unenforceable, because no woman should be forced to give up a child based on a surrender statement signed prior to conception or birth.

The Committee to Defend Reproductive Rights (CDRR) was founded in 1977 in response to the Hyde Amendment, which cut off federal funds for abortion. Since that time, it has become an advocate for reproductive freedom both in the courtroom and in the public sphere. CDRR has focused attention on sterilization abuse, the impact of prenatal diagnosis and other technological intervention during pregnancy on women's rights, and court-mandated interventions that pit the fetus against the mother. Another concern of CDRR is that where reproductive services are offered, access be guaranteed regardless of the woman's marital status or sexual orientation.

Despite the impressive array of groups that are hostile toward new reproductive applications and fearful of their impact on society, one should never underestimate the influence of the medical establishment on public policy. In combination with a politically powerful research community that carries with it substantial momentum, the expanding commercial industry of human reproduction, with its huge economic stake, represents a formidable political force in favor of the proliferation and diffusion of these technologies. As reproduction becomes more medicalized and, thus, solidly the domain of the medical establishment, much to the disapproval of feminists, it will be increasingly difficult to curtail diffusion of evermore sophisticated intervention techniques.

The supportive interests, however, go well beyond those persons whose careers or economic interests rest on these technologies. There is no doubt that these technologies offer benefits to many persons. It is not surprising, therefore, that groups have been established specifically to support expanded access to these innovations. Millions of couples are potential users of these techniques and many of them are likely to support research and development in this area. RESOLVE, Inc., was established in 1974 as a support and referral group for infertile couples. Its national headquarters and chapters in most states have been active in lobbying for increased reproductive-mediating services and for public funding of IVF and other techniques. Likewise, Surrogates by Choice is a national association of surrogate mothers established to protect the right of women to play that role. The rapid growth of these organizations also demonstrates that there is substantial untapped public support for these technologies. As new techniques for sex preselection, genetic testing and diagnosis, and genetic therapy emerge, many other groups are likely to lend support to those applications that heighten the interests of their constituencies.

Political Feasibility

Interest-group activity in reproductive issues will continue to cut across traditional social and political lines in American society. Due to the complexity of the problems raised by these technologies and the value conflicts they produce, future alignments of groups will differ substantially from those on other political issues. This makes it highly unlikely that either major political party will be able to adopt a strong policy stand on reproductive technologies without risking the loss of substantial elements in their bases of support. At the same time, the high stakes involved in policy decisions concerning genetic intervention will accentuate group activity and magnify conflict among the interests.

The political feasibility of any reproductive policy is dependent on the reaction of these many conflicting stakeholders. This situation, of course, is no different than for any other policy area. However, because reproduction is such a politically sensitive issue, and one that can easily escalate to a pivotal campaign issue, political feasibility analysis here must carefully weigh the extent to which the support or opposition can mobilize broader public support and media sympathy, which—to date—favor the technologies. To a large extent, the intensity of the response of any group depends on the perceived threat of the proposed action to its interests. It is crucial, then, that policy makers be aware of the issues that are of most concern to the various parties and that they explicitly frame the policy so as to anticipate the problems and deal with them prospectively.

FRAMING A CONSENSUAL BASE FOR REPRODUCTIVE POLICY

To date, the debate over reproductive technologies, and indeed the thrust of this book, has focused on the conflicts and policy problems they raise. This is natural because policy issues arise only in conflict situations—if there is no disagreement, there is no issue. Pluralism, however, elevates conflict at the expense of building a consensus, as each of many groups acts to protect its perceived interests. Although the degree of conflict over these interventions cannot be overstated, the result of the political process in the United States is to obscure potential bases of agreement while aggrandizing conflicts over values, the distribution of resources, and so forth. As each group builds its case, it naturally focuses attention on those aspects of the interventions that support its stand, thus heightening the controversy and reducing the possibility of real dialogue.

Although the sensitive issues raised by human reproductive technology will never be fully resolved, any rational policy must build on common ground. Despite the deep divisions among the combating forces, there are some bases upon which a consensus might be developed. People will continue to differ as to the best means of achieving these goals as well as to the specific criteria that define them, but consensual support in these areas would go a long way to modulate the intensity of the debate over reproductive policy. These areas of common ground in the United States include a desire for:

1. The best possible health for children
2. The reduction of infertility
3. The minimization of risk or misuse of reproductive intervention
4. The maximization of individual freedom and choice
5. The maintenance of social order
6. The best possible existence for future generations.

If some agreement can be reached on these goals, specific technological applications can be judged in light of their implications for achieving these societal objectives. After discussing each of these factors in turn, a framework for analyzing an array of reproductive innovations is presented.

Healthy Children

No rational parents would prefer that their child be unhealthy. Moreover, most parents would go to considerable expense and effort to ensure as healthy and happy a life possible for their child. Therefore, to oppose a policy on the grounds that it contributes to the health of our progeny seems unthinkable. Although a small minority of the population rejects interventions designed to reduce ill health, their major opposition would seem to be a function of the current state of the art. For example, right-to-life groups often oppose prenatal diagnosis because they argue, correctly, that it currently results in elimination of the affected being rather than treatment for the disease.

Certainly the goal of healthy children is undermined if the means to that end is to terminate the lives of potential unhealthy children. It is quite a different matter, however, to use the same prenatal diagnostic techniques to identify a fetus with a genetic disorder and then apply therapy to overcome the problem. Current developments in fetal surgery and promised advances in gene therapy illustrate such an approach.

One criterion that can be used to evaluate a technological innovation, then, is whether it contributes to the health of an identifiable potential child. If it does, the burden of proof is on those who would block its use. For instance, the use of AID by a woman to circumvent her husband's hereditary disease or of egg donation to accomplish the same end for a woman carrier would fulfill this criterion of protecting the health of her potential progeny. In contrast, the use of AID to overcome infertility or for eugenic purposes would have to be justified on other grounds.

A vexing question that will intensify as more precise diagnostic and therapeutic capacities emerge is where to draw the line on what is defined as the "health" of the child. Certainly, most uses of sex selection and many potential applications of genetic diagnosis and therapy are preference- rather than health-based decisions. As DNA probes and other techniques develop that eventually give parents the opportunity to select for specific characteristics that, in effect, design their version of the "perfect" child, the line between healthy child and preferred child will become even more obscured. The growing demand for human growth therapy by parents of short, but not hormonally deficient, children raises difficult ethical dilemmas, because it is a reflection of a cultural stigma against short people, not a health problem in the traditional sense (Lantos, Siegler, and Cuttler 1989). As the technical means to ameliorate shortness and other preference-based characteristics are found, even greater stigma will be attached to the persons who are unlucky enough to share them. Under these circumstances, it becomes even more critical to distinguish between those interventions that actually lead to healthier children and those that simply give parents more control over their children's physical attributes.

Reducing Infertility

Whatever one's views about specific techniques or preferred strategies, the goal of reducing infertility undoubtedly enjoys consensual support. Parenthood and the family idea have considerable support in the U.S. and infertility is viewed as a condition that should be amenable to technological intervention. Moreover, as infertility increases and more persons are directly or indirectly affected, demands to reduce infertility will heighten. The rapidly growing use of AID, IVF, and other TMRs clearly reflects this desire to overcome infertility.

One of the dangers of an overdependence on TMRs to "fix" infertility problems is its tendency to deflect the use of resources to find the causes of infertility and to then prevent them. Table 8.1 illustrates why preventive strategies are more likely to succeed than attempts to treat infertility. The broad range of factors predisposing individuals toward infertility suggests that in the long run prevention makes sense. Even at the present time, among infertile couples seeking treatment, 85 to 90 percent are treated with conventional counseling, medical therapy, or surgical therapy (OTA, 1988:7). This also raises a question of the large potential costs associated with proliferation of curative reproductive services when compared to the costs of a preventive approach. Although disagreement will continue as to which strategy to overcome infertility is preferable, it is probable that both are necessary. Therefore, it is likely that the use of TMRs to overcome fertility problems for persons otherwise unable to procreate will serve as another basis for their support. Despite continuing antagonism by some groups toward all reproductive technologies, opposition is likely to be muted for those applications that circumvent infertility.

Minimization of Risk and Misuse

Whether one favors or opposes diffusion of reproductive intervention techniques, it is likely that he or she will agree that, when

TABLE 8.1. Prevention of Infertility

Factors predisposing individuals toward infertility and preventive steps available

Sexually transmitted diseases (STDs) and pelvic inflammatory disease (PID):
- Careful selection of possible sexual partners. Health education to discourage unprotected sexual encounters. Monogamy. Forthright inquiry and check of sexual partners for risks of STDs.
- Contraception by means of condoms. Use condoms routinely with new sex partner. Media campaign to encourage condom use.
- Periodic screening for STDs, if sexually active; STDs in both males and females are commonly asymptomatic.
- Changes in societal attitudes about STDs to lessen stigma of diagnostic examination for them.
- Recognize findings of STDs and seek medical care. Ensure that correct treatment is given for yourself and partner, with followup.
- Media campaign to encourage men and women with genital discharge to be checked for STDs.
- Rapid, adequate management of PID to reduce risk of sequelae.

Pelvic infections after birth, abortion, surgery, or invasive diagnostic testing:
- Ensure that optimally safe birth and surgical services are available.
- Use prophylactic antibiotics in high-risk situations to prevent infection.

Exercise, poor nutrition, and stress:
- Recognize that regular strenuous exercise (i.e., exceeding 60 minutes daily), rapid weight loss, low body fat, and stress may cause decreased fertility. Women are at higher risk than men.

Smoking, environmental toxins, and drugs:
- Smoking, as well as other substance abuse, reduces reproductive potential and should be avoided. Environmental exposures are inadequately studied, but appear more common in males. Semen analysis can be performed.

used, risk must be minimized, and conversely, benefits maximized in any application. Although opponents might be hesitant to express this view out of fear of undermining their stand against all applications, given the inevitability of escalation of their use, those techniques which pose minimum risk and maximum benefit are likely to appreciate broad public support. In contrast, those techniques that entail a substantial risk to any of the parties, including

Endometriosis:
- If strong family history for endometriosis exists, consider oral contraception and possible specific endometriosis suppression. Oral contraceptives may suppress endometriosis even in those not at high risk.
- Early diagnosis and treatment in symptomatic women. Conservative surgical approaches.

Cryptorchidism and varicocele:
- Undescended, especially intra-abdominal, testes should be treated as promptly as possible. Benefits of surveillance and treatment of varicocele are controversial.

Chemotherapy and radiation:
- Risks of gonadal damage must be considered and, if appropriate, gamete collection or protection of the gonads should be performed.

Intercurrent illnesses:
- Many acute and chronic diseases cause anovulation or decreased spermatogenesis. Prevention of these effects is by treatment of the primary disease.

Inadequate knowledge of reproduction:
- Ensure that information on reproduction is available from parents, schools, clergy, and other sources.

Inadequate medical treatment:
- Couples with difficulty conceiving should educate themselves about fertility and seek specialized care before infertility is prolonged.

Lack of perspective about reproduction:
- Discuss family life with parents, peers, and professionals. Formulate life plan that allows adequate time for reproductive goals.

SOURCE: Office of Technology Assessment, 1988, p. 86.

the potential child, or that threaten existing social institutions such as the family are less likely to be supported by society as a whole.

The entrenchment of the technological imperative in the U.S. value system precludes the likelihood of highly restrictive policies regarding reproductive technologies in general. More likely is an intensified emphasis on consumer protection, reduction of risk, and regulation to ensure the safety and efficacy of reproductive services. If a particular application can withstand public scrutiny regarding its risk and it promises appreciable benefits in advancing the health of children or overcoming infertility, broad support is probable.

Individual Freedom and Choice

Underlying the potential consensual approval of techniques that bear minimal risk is a widespread support for the U.S. regime and for continuance of social order. If the public perceives a technology as a threat to existing social institutions and community values, it faces considerable condemnation. If, on the other hand, a reproductive technology is viewed as extending these values and structures, acceptance is all but guaranteed.

At the core of American political culture is the value of individual freedom, which is often operationalized through the concept of rights. As described earlier, procreative autonomy especially is highly valued in the U.S. and has enjoyed a broad interpretation by the Supreme Court over the last half century. As a result, it is very difficult to preclude the availability and individual use of any technique that expands individual choice. The problem in determining this remains, however, that every technique can be applied variously either to expand or constrain individual choice. Clear distinctions, therefore, must be made between free and informed voluntary applications and involuntary or coerced applications. While consensual support is likely for the former, it is improbable for the latter.

A related issue that must be faced by policy makers is that of payment. If reproduction is a fundamental human right as the Court has ruled, it is unfair to deny these services to persons who cannot afford them. Because of the special status given procreation, it is difficult to justify inequities in access to the technologies that extend that right. Although the costs of such guaranteed access promise to be considerable, there are likely to be escalating demands for public funding of those applications that extend procreative choice. Clearly, this is one area where the economic realities of scarce resources come into conflict with political expediency arising out of group demands for governmental support for reproductive services. It also exemplifies the urgency of establishing a national dialogue on how best to allocate health care resources and demonstrates the inherent conflict between individual needs and societal priorities.

Benefits to Future Generations

One extension of the goal of ensuring healthy children is to use technologies in ways that are likely to benefit, not harm, future generations. Although disagreement will continue to exist over how to conceptualize benefits to remote, and to some extent unimaginable, humans, interventions perceived as irreversibly harmful to future generations, those that preclude their choice, will fail to achieve broad support no matter how attractive they are to some individuals now living. In contrast, reproductive technologies that are not viewed as threats to the quality of life of future humans are likely to be supported. Again, given our propensity to depend on technology, the burden of proof will be on those interests which oppose deployment.

Of all the areas of possible consensus regarding reproductive intervention introduced here, concern for the future is least developed even though the major impact of the decisions we make today surrounding human genetics and reproduction will fall on future inhabitants. As discussed earlier, considerable effort is needed to refocus the debate over reproductive intervention to include recognition of the long-term implications of our actions in the present.

Consensual Goal Criteria for Reproductive Policy

Table 8.2 is not intended to be a definitive categorization or judgment of specific techniques based on these consensual goal criteria. Rather, it is presented solely to illustrate one type of analysis that should accompany efforts to frame a workable reproductive policy. At best, this scheme offers a starting point for a more in-depth assessment of each technology. Political feasibility eventually depends on the degree of support that a policy option can engender from the relevant interest groups and attentive publics. If a technology is congruent with these areas of broad societal agreement, however, the likelihood of its approval is enhanced.

In table 8.2, a plus sign (+) is assigned to those interventions that are likely to achieve consensual approval for the appropriate goal. A question mark (?) is assigned to those techniques whose fit is presently questionable, either for technological or social reasons, while a minus (−) score represents those applications that are unlikely to gain support for each item. In several cases the designation "NA" is used to represent that that technique is not applicable to that goal. Those applications which score mostly "+" are least likely to have trouble gaining public acceptance, while those scoring " − " face significant obstacles.

The numerous scores of "?" in table 8.2 demonstrate the current high levels of uncertainty and, more importantly, the need for intensive analyses of the social consequences of most types of human genetic and reproductive mediation. Many of those labeled "?" arguably could be scored " + " and undoubtedly will, upon closer

TABLE 8.2. Technology Compliance to Consensual Goal Criteria

	Healthy Children	Reduce Infertility	Minimize Risk	Maximize Individual Choice	Benefit Future Humans
AID	+	+	+	+	?
IVF	?	+	?	+	?
GIFT	?	+	?	+	?
Embryo Lavage	?	+	?	+	?
Egg Donation	?	+	?	+	?
Embryo Donation	?	+	?	+	?
SM	?	+	?	?	?
Sex Preselection	?	NA	?	+	?
Amniocentesis	+	NA	+	?	+
CVS	?	NA	?	?	+
Ultrasound	+	NA	+	?	+
Embryo Research	?	?	?	?	?
Fetal Surgery	+	NA	?	+	?
Somatic GT	?	?	?	?	?
Germline GT	?	?	?	?	?
Sterilization					
voluntary	?	NA	+	+	+
involuntary	?	NA	+	−	?
Subdermal Implants	?	NA	?	+	+
RU 486	?	NA	?	+	?
Prenatal Care	+	+	+	+	+
Preventive Medicine	+	+	+	−	+

study. Although full agreement on the values assigned here is unlikely, all but the most confirmed opponents of reproductive technologies should find the variation in support, based on compliance with these criteria, meaningful.

CONCLUSIONS

Although the ethical issues surrounding human genetic and reproductive technologies have received considerable attention over the past decade and are integral to any attempts at political resolution, this book focused instead on questions concerning the role of government in reproductive research and application. What is the proper role of government in matters of reproductive choice, which public mechanisms are best suited to handle these issues, and who ought to be responsible for making the difficult policy decisions that are essential? It demonstrated the intricacy and scope of the policy problems inherent in reproductive intervention. Unfortunately, it also illustrates the lack of ready solutions and the understandable difficulties that policy makers have in coping with these issues.

On the critical question of who ought to make these hard policy decisions for society, the conclusion here is that the dialogue must be expanded to comprise as much of the citizenry as possible. Within the context of the American political scene, this should include attempts to enlarge that portion of the public attentive to reproductive and genetic issues. Inclusion of the attentive public in an open dialogue concerning goals and priorities is most crucial at this point. A permanent commission-type body along the lines of the temporary President's Commission for the Study of Ethical Problems, but with a focus on reproductive issues, would represent a meaningful beginning point. The recommendation for a continuous review of reproductive and genetic technology goes beyond the Commission's own recommendation (1982:79) that the development of genetic technology "will require periodic reassessment as greater knowledge is gained." The creation of such a body would have the advantage of relieving elected officials of these no-win issues, but it should supplement, not replace, the establishment of a long-range planning mechanism along the lines suggested by Milbrath. Only through an institution of that type can we exercise our responsibility to future generations.

Technology assessment, political feasibility analysis, and other methods for analyzing alternative courses of action must be utilized by appropriate agencies of government, though no one approach can be relied on exclusively. Despite relevant disclaimers by some observers, it is crucial that assessment be initiated at as early a stage as possible in the development of each technique, before it is widely diffused. It is essential that we, as a society, soon establish priorities as to which lines of research should be pursued and which applications should be promoted. Although no quick and easy solutions are possible, and even the long-term resolution of these problems remains doubtful, considerable effort must be expended to clarify the social policy dimensions of reproductive technology and place them in the broader social context. Successful channeling of these technologies into "socially acceptable" directions requires a vigorous and cohesive commitment on the part of policy makers, the research community, and those members of the public concerned enough about the future of reproductive choice to become informed if given the opportunity. Decisions made now are likely to delimit the options available to future generations as well as to constrain or extend the choices available to existing generations.

In spite of the magnitude of the problems in human procreation facing our society and the seeming inability of existing political institutions to grapple with the rapidity of the technological and social change they engender, these issues are so critical to the continuance of our way of life, or to achievement of a more preferred one, that no effort should be spared in working toward their resolution. While acrimonious political conflict is bound to accompany any attempts to establish social policy (including regulation) in human reproduction, the stakes are becoming too high to continue on the path of least resistance.

We urgently need an intensive, creative, public dialogue on reproductive technologies. The issues we currently face will not dissipate, or resolve themselves. Rather, they are certain to become more complicated, as evermore sophisticated and intrusive reproductive interventions are dispersed across an ever-expanding proportion of the population. Building on the areas of consensus discussed here, we have hope of reaching a manageable, yet always tenuous, foundation of agreement on social priorities and, thus, a meaningful policy base for regulating human reproductive technologies. Human procreation is too valuable an endeavor to leave to the vagaries of conventional politics, nor can we afford to let it be a captive of the workings of the marketplace. More than in any past era, we now hold within our grasp both our destiny and that of future generations. Although the move is as yet ours, fast approaching is that time where we will lose the capacity to define these technologies in our own terms. At that point, it will be too late to exercise human control.

APPENDIX A

International Activities in Human Reproductive Technology: Selected Reports, Regulations, and Laws

AUSTRALIA

1985 Senate Standing Committee on Constitutional and Legal Affairs *(IVF and the Status of Children)*.

1985 Family Law Council of the Attorney General's Office *(Creating Children: A Uniform Approach to the Law and Practice of Reproductive Technology in Australia)*.

1985 Guidelines of the National Health and Medical Research Council *(Statement on Human Experimentation and Supplementary Notes)*.

1986. Select Committee on the Human Embryo Experimentation Bill *(Human Embryo Experimentation in Australia)*.

New South Wales

1986 Law Reform Commission *(Artificial Conception Report 1: Human Artificial Insemination).*
1987 LRC *(Artificial Conception Discussion Paper 2: In Vitro Fertilization).*
1988 LRC *(Artificial Conception Report 2: In Vitro Fertilization).*
1984 Artificial Conception Act.

Queensland

1984 Report of the Special Committee Appointed by the Queensland Government to Enquire into Laws Relating to Artificial Insemination, In Vitro Fertilization, and Other Related Matters.

South Australia

1984 Report of the Working Party on In Vitro Fertilization and Artificial Insemination by Donor.
1984 Family Relationships Amendment Act.

Tasmania

1985 Committee to Investigate Artificial Conception and Related Matters *(Final Report).*

Victoria

1982 Committee to Consider the Social, Ethical, and Legal Issues Arising from In Vitro Fertilization The Waller Commission *(Interim Report).*
1984 CCS *(Report on Donor Gametes in IVF).*
1985 CCS *(Report on the Disposition of Embryos Produced by In Vitro Fertilization).*
1984 The Status of Children *(Amendment)* Act.
1984 The Infertility *(Medical Procedures)* Act.

Western Australia

1984 Committee to Enquire into the Social, Legal, and Ethical Issues Relating to In Vitro Fertilization and Its Supervision *(Interim Report).*
1986 *(Report).*

AUSTRIA

1986 Ministry of Sciences and Research *(The Fundamental Aspects of Genetics and Reproductive Biology)*.

BRAZIL

1957 Code of Medical Rules *(Article 53 prohibits AID)*.

CANADA

1981 Advisory Committee to the Minister of National Health and Welfare *(Storage and Utilization of Human Sperm)*.
1987 Medical Research Council *(Discussion Draft of Revised Guidelines on Research Involving Human Subjects of the Medical Research Council of Canada)*.

Alberta

1976 Institute of Law Research and Reform *(Status of Children)*.

British Columbia

1975 Royal Commission on Family and Children's Law *(Ninth Report of the Royal Commission on Family and Children's Law: Artificial Insemination)*.

Ontario

1985 Law Reform Commission *(Report on Human Artificial Reproduction and Related Matters)*.

Saskatchewan

1987 Law Reform Commission *(Proposals for a Human Artificial Insemination Act)*.

COUNCIL OF EUROPE

1986 Ad Hoc Committee of Experts on Progress in the Biomedical Sciences (CAHBI) *(Provisional Principles on the Techniques of Human Artificial Procreation and Certain Procedures Carried Out on Embryos in Connection with Those Techniques)*.

CZECHOSLOVAKIA

1982 Family Law *(Article 52-2 legitimizes AID children).*

DENMARK

1984 Government Committee Report *(Ethical Problems with Egg Transplantation, AID, and Research on Embryos).*

FEDERAL REPUBLIC OF GERMANY

1985 Federal Ministry for Research and Technology and Ministry of Justice, The Benda Report *(IVF, Genome Analysis, and Gene Therapy).*
1987 Federal-State Working Group *(Interim Report: Reproductive Medicine).*
1987 Ad Hoc Commission to German Parliament *(Risk Assessment of Genetic Engineering).*

FRANCE

1986 Comite Consultatif National d'Ethique pour les Sciences (CCNE) *(Journés Annuelles d'Ethique, Sommaire).*

GREECE

1983 Civil Code *(Article 1471/2-2, Law 1329).*

INTERNATIONAL LAW ASSOCIATION

1986 *International Mechanisms of Protection of the Human Person and Reproductive Technology.*

ISRAEL

1987 Ministry of Health *(Public Health (Extra-corporeal Fertilization) Regulations of 1987).*

ITALY

1985 Ministry of Health Committee *(Santosuossa Report)*.

LIBYA

Criminal Code *(Articles 304A and 304B outlaw artificial insemination)*.

NETHERLANDS

1986 Health Council of the Netherlands *(Report on Reproductive Technologies)*.

NEW ZEALAND

1985 Law Reform Division, Department of Justice *(New Birth Technologies: An Issues Paper on AID, IVF, and Surrogate Motherhood)*.
1986 LRC *(New Birth Technologies: A Summary of Submissions Received on the Issues Paper)*.

NORWAY

1983 Council of Medical Research *(Directives in Ethical Matters for Artificial Insemination and In Vitro Fertilization)*.
1987 Act #68. Regulates AID and IVF.

SOUTH AFRICA

1986 Department of National Health and Population Development *(Regulations Regarding the Artificial Insemination of Persons)*.

SPAIN

1986 Report of Special Commission for the Study of Human In Vitro Fertilization and Artificial Insemination.

Eisbrenner v. Stanley, 106 Mi.A. 357, 308 N.W.2d 209 (1981)

Eisenstadt v. Baird, 405 U.S. 438 (1972)

Ellis v. Sherman, No. J26052 (Pa. 1984)

Gleitman v. Cosgrove, 49 N.J. 22, 227 A.2d 689 (1967)

Graham v. Pima City, Pima City Super. Ct., No. 190297 (Jan. 18, 1983)

Griswold v. Connecticut, 381 U.S. 479, 484 (1965)

Harbeson v. Parke-Davis, 98 Wash.2d 460, 656 P.2d 483 (1983)

In re Baby M., 537 A.2d 1227 (N.J. 1988)

Margaret S. v. Edwards, 794 F.2d 994 (La. 1986)

Nelson v. Krusen, 635 S.W.2d 582 (Tex. 1982)

People v. Sorenson, 668 Cal.2d 280, 437 P.2d 495 (1968)

Procanik v. Cillo, N.J. Sup. Ct. No. A-89 (1984)

Roe v. Wade 410 U.S. 113 (1973)

Schroeder v. Perkel, 87 N.J. 53 (S.C.N.J. July 15, 1981)

Skinner v. Oklahoma, 316 U.S. 535 (1942)

Smith v. Hartigan, 556 F. Supp. 157 (N.D.Ill. 1983)

Strnad v. Strnad, 190 Misc. 786, 78 N.Y.S.2d 390 (Sup. Ct. 1948)

Surrogate Parenting Associates, Inc. v. Commonwealth ex rel. Armstrong, 704 S.W.2d 209 (Ky. 1986)

Thornburgh v. American College of Obstetricians and Gynecologists, 476 U.S. 747 (1986)

Webster v. Reproductive Health Services, 57 U.S. L.W. 5023 (July 3, 1989)

Zepeda v. Zepeda, 41 Ill. App.2d 240, 190 N.E.2d 849 (1963)

BIBLIOGRAPHY

Adams, Melissa M., Godfred P. Oakley, and James S. Marks. 1982. "Maternal Age and Births in the 1980s." *JAMA* 247:493–498.

Affandi, Biran, Joedo Prihartono, Firmin Lubis, Hermini Sutedi, and R.S. Samil. 1987. "Insertion and Removal of NORPLANT Contraceptive Implants by Physicians and Nonphysicians in an Indonesian Clinic." *Studies on Family Planning* 18(5):302–306.

Almond, Gabriel A. 1960. *The American People and Foreign Policy*. New York: Praeger.

American Association of Tissue Banks. 1984. *Standards for Tissue Banking*. Rockville, Md.: AATB.

American College of Obstetricians and Gynecologists. 1984. "Human In Vitro Fertilization and Embryo Placement." Committee Statement (April).

American Fertility Society. 1986a. "Ethical Considerations of the New Reproductive Technologies." *Fertility and Sterility* 46(3):Supp. 1.

——1986b. "New Guidelines for the Use of Semen Donor Insemination." *Fertility and Sterility* 46(4):Supp. 2.

———1988a. "Revised New Guidelines for the Use of Semen-Donor Insemination." *Fertility and Sterility* 49(2):211.

———1988b. "Minimal Standards for Gamete Intrafallopian Transfer (GIFT)." *Fertility and Sterility* 50(1):20.

American Medical News, March 18, 1988, p. 11.

Anderson, W. French. 1984. "Prospects for Human Gene Therapy." *Science* 226:401–409.

Andrews, Lori B. 1981. "Embryo Technology." *Parents* (May):pp. 63–70.

———1984. *New Conceptions: A Consumer's Guide to the Newest Infertility Treatments*. New York: St. Martin's Press.

———1986. "Legal and Ethical Aspects of New Reproductive Technologies." *Clinical Obstetrics and Gynecology* 29(1):190–204.

Annas, George J. 1980. "Fathers Anonymous: Beyond the Best Interests of the Donor." *Family Law Quarterly* 14(1):1–13.

———1984. "Surrogate Embryo Transfer: The Perils of Patenting." *Hastings Center Report* 14(3):25–26.

Arditti, Rita. 1985. "Review Essay: Reducing Women to Matter." *Women's Studies International Forum* 8(6):577–582.

Arehart-Treichel, J. 1980. "Questioning the New Genetics." *Science News* 116:155–156.

Association for Voluntary Surgical Contraception. 1988. "Current Status of Sterilization Laws Regarding Mentally Retarded Persons." Mimeo.

Attanasio, John B. 1986. "The Constitutionality of Regulating Human Genetic Engineering: Where Procreative Liberty and Equal Opportunity Collide." *University of Chicago Law Review* 53(4):1274–1342.

Baltimore, David 1983. "Can Genetic Science Backfire?" 'That's the Chance We Take.' " *U.S. News and World Report*, March 28, pp. 52–53.

Barkay, John, and H. Zuckerman. 1980. "The Role of Cryobanking in Artificial Insemination." In G. David and W. S. Price, eds., *Human Artificial Insemination and Semen Preservation*. New York: Plenum Press.

Barnes, Deborah M. 1988. "Schizophrenia Genetics a Mixed Bag." *Science* 242(November19):1009.

Beckwith, Jon. 1976. "Social and Political Uses of Genetics in the United States: Past and Present." *Annals of the New York Academy of Sciences* 265:46–58.

Begent, R. H. J. 1980. "Semen Storage for Patients with Cancer." In David W. Richardson et al., eds., *Frozen Human Semen*. Amsterdam: Martinus Nijhoff.

Beiner, Ronald. 1988. "Introduction." In Richard B. Day, Ronald Beiner, and Joseph Masciulli, eds., *Democratic Theory and Technological Society*. Armonk, N.Y.: M. E. Sharpe.

Benacerraf, Beryl R., Rebecca Gelman, and Fredric D. Frigoletto. 1987. "Sonographic Identification of Second-Trimester Fetuses with Down's Syndrome." *JAMA* 317(22):1371–1376.

Berkowitz, Richard L., Lauren Lynch, Usha Chitkara, Isabelle A. Wilkins,

Karen E. Mehalek, and Emanuel Alvarez. 1988. "Selective Reduction of Multifetal Pregnancies in the First Trimester." *New England Journal of Medicine* 318(16):1043–1047.

Best, James M. 1973. *Public Opinion: Micro and Macro*. Homewood, Ill.: Dorsey Press.

Biggers, John D. 1981. "In Vitro Fertilization and Embryo Transfer in Humans." *New England Journal of Medicine* 304:336–342.

Bird, K. 1982. "Surrogate Motherhood: Hers? Yours? Ours?" *California Lawyer* 2(2):21–25.

Bishop, Jerry E., and Michael Waldholz. 1986. "The Search for a Perfect Child." *Wall Street Journal*, March 19.

Blank, Robert H. 1981. *The Political Implications of Human Genetic Technology*. Boulder: Westview Press.

——1985. "The Wrongful Life Dilemma: An Update." *Bioethics Reporter*. Fredericksburg, Md.: University Publications of America.

——1986. "Emerging Notions of Women's Rights and Responsibilities During Gestation." *Journal of Legal Medicine* 7(4):441–469.

Boldt, Jeffrey. 1988. "Micromanipulation in Human Reproductive Technology." *Fertility and Sterility* 50(2):213–215.

Bonnicksen, Andrea L. 1985. "The Policy of Alternative Conception: Looking to the States." Paper presented at the Annual Meeting of the American Political Science Association, New Orleans, August 29.

——1989. *In Vitro Fertilization: Building Policy from Laboratories to Legislatures*. New York: Columbia University Press.

Bonnicksen, Andrea L. and Robert H. Blank. 1988. "The Government and In Vitro Fertilization (IVF): Views of IVF Directors." *Fertility and Sterility* 49 (3):396–398.

Botkin, Jeffrey R. 1988. "The Legal Concept of Wrongful Life." *JAMA* 259(10):1541–1545.

Brahams, Diana. 1987. "The Hasty British Ban on Commercial Surrogacy." *Hastings Center Report* 17(1):16–19.

Brewer, Gary D., and Peter deLeon. 1983. *The Foundations of Policy Analysis*. Homewood, Ill.: Dorsey Press.

Brophy, Katie M. 1982. "A Surrogate Mother Contract to Bear a Child." *Journal of Family Law* 20:263–281.

Buchanan, Cathy, and Elizabeth W. Prior. 1984. "Bureaucrats and Babies: Government Regulation of the Supply of Genetic Material." *The Economic Record* (September), pp. 222–230.

Capron, Alexander M. 1979. "Tort Liability in Genetic Counseling." *Columbia Law Review* 79:619–684.

——1980. "The Wrong of 'Wrongful Life.' " In Aubrey Milunsky and George J. Annas, eds., *Genetics and the Law II*. New York: Plenum Press.

Carey, William D. 1982. "Observations: Racing the Time Constants." In A.H. Teich and R. Thornton, eds., *Science, Technology, and the Issues of the Eighties: Policy Outlook*. Boulder: Westview Press.

Carmen, Ira. 1986. *Cloning and the Constitution*. Madison: University of Wisconsin Press.

Carson, Sandra Ann. 1988. "Sex Selection: The Ultimate in Family Planning." *Fertility and Sterility* 50(1):16–19.

Chadwick, Ruth F., ed. 1987. *Ethics, Reproduction, and Genetic Control*. New York: Croom Helm.

Chapman, J. 1979. "What Are Your Odds in the Prenatal Gamble?" *Legal Aspects of Medical Practice* 31:34.

Chorover, Steven L. 1980. *From Genesis to Genocide: The Meaning of Human Nature and the Power of Behavior Control*. Cambridge: MIT Press.

Coates, Joseph F. 1971. "Technology Assessment: The Benefits, The Costs, The Consequences." *Futurist* 5:1060–1067.

——— 1978. "What is a Policy Issue?" In Kenneth R. Hammond, ed., *Judgment and Decision in Public Policy Formation*. Boulder: Westview Press.

Cohen, Jacques, Gary W. De Vane, Carlene W. Elsner, and Carole B. Fehilly. 1988. "Cryopreservation of Zygotes and Early Cleaved Human Embryos." *Fertility and Sterility* 49(2):283–289.

Collingridge, David. 1980. *The Social Control of Technology*. New York: St. Martin's Press.

Cooper, Jay M. and Robert M. Houck. 1983. "Study Protocol, Criteria, and Complications of the Silicone Plug Procedure." In Gerald I. Zatuchni et al., eds., *Female Transcervical Sterilization*. Philadelphia: Harper and Row.

Corea, Gina. 1985. *The Mother Machine: Reproductive Technologies from Artificial Insemination to Artificial Wombs*. New York: Harper and Row.

——— 1985a. *The Hidden Malpractice: How American Medicine Mistreats Women*, 2d ed. New York: Harper and Row.

Council on Scientific Affairs, American Medical Association. 1982. "Maternal Serum Alpha Fetoprotein Monitoring." *JAMA* 247:1478.

Curie-Cohen, N., L. Luttrell, and S. Shapiro. 1979. "Current Practice of Artificial Insemination by Donor in the United States." *New England Journal of Medicine* 300:585–590.

Dahl, Robert A. 1970. *After The Revolution*. New Haven: Yale University Press.

——— 1985. *Controlling Nuclear Weapons: Democracy Versus Guardianship*. Syracuse: Syracuse University Press.

DeCherney, Alan H., and G. S. Berkowitz. 1982. "Female Fecundity and Age." *New England Journal of Medicine* 306:424–426.

Department of Health, Education and Welfare, National Institutes of Health. 1979. *Antenatal Diagnosis: Predictors of Hereditary Disease or Congenital Defects*. Washington, D.C.: U.S. Government Printing Office.

Department of Health and Social Security. 1986. *Legislation on Infertility Services and Embryo Research: A Consultation Paper*. London: Her Majesty's Stationery Office.

Devine, Donald J. 1970. *The Attentive Public: Polyarchical Democracy*. Chicago: Rand McNally.

——1972. *The Political Culture of the United States*. Boston: Little, Brown.

Dickson, David. 1988. "Europe Split on Embryo Research" *Science* 242 (November): 1117–1118.

Dresser, Rebecca. 1985. "Social Justice in New Reproductive Techniques." In Aubrey Milunsky and George J. Annas, eds., *Genetics and the Law III*. New York: Plenum Press.

Drucker, Peter F. 1981. "New Technology: Predicting Its Impact." In Albert H. Teich, ed., *Technology and Man's Future*. 3rd ed. New York: St. Martin's Press.

Edwards, R.G. 1974. "Fertilization of Human Eggs In Vitro: Morals, Ethics and the Law." *Quarterly Review of Biology* 49(1):3–26.

Elias, Sherman, Joe Leigh Simpson, Alice O. Martin, Rudy E. Sabbagha, Albert B. Gerbie, and Louis G. Keith. 1985. "Chorionic Villus Sampling for First-Trimester Prenatal Diagnosis." *American Journal of Obstetrics and Gynecology* 152:204–213.

Ethics Advisory Board. 1979. *HEW Support of Research Involving Human In Vitro Fertilization and Embryo Transfer*. Washington, D.C.: U.S. Government Printing Office.

Etzioni, Amitai. 1973. *Genetic Fix: The Next Technological Revolution*. New York: Harper and Row.

Feinberg, Joel. 1974. *Doing and Deserving: Essays on the Theory of Responsibility*. Princeton: Princeton University Press.

Ferkiss, Victor. 1978. "Technology Assessment and Appropriate Technology." *National Forum* (Fall), pp. 3–7.

Field, Martha A. 1988. *Surrogate Motherhood*. Cambridge: Harvard University Press.

Flannery, D. M. et al. 1978. "Legal Issues Concerning In Vitro Fertilization." Paper prepared for Ethics Advisory Board.

Fletcher, Joseph F. 1974. *The Ethics of Genetic Control: Ending Reproductive Roulette*. Garden City: Doubleday.

Forbes, H. D. 1988. "Dahl, Democracy and Technology." In Richard B. Day, Ronald Beiner, and Joseph Masciulli, eds., *Democratic Theory and Technological Society*. Armonk, N.Y.: M. E. Sharpe.

Forrest, Jacqueline D. and Stanley K. Henshaw. 1983. "What U.S. Women Think and Do About Contraception." *Family Planning Perspectives* 15(4):157–166.

Frankel, Charles. 1976. "The Specter of Eugenics." In N. Ostheimer and John Ostheimer, eds. *Life or Death: Who Controls?* New York: Springer.

Frankel, Mark S. 1976. "Human-Semen Banking: Social and Public Policy Issues." *Man and Medicine* 1(4):289–309.

——1979. "Artificial Insemination and Semen Cryobanking: Health and Safety Concerns.." *Legal-Medical Quarterly* 3(2):93–100.

Frederickson, Donald S. 1978. "The Public Governance of Science." *Man and Medicine* 3(2):77–88.

Freeman, David M. 1974. *Technology and Society: Issues in Assessment, Conflict and Choice*. Chicago: Rand McNally.

Freeman, Ellen W., Andrea S. Boxer, Karl Rickels, Richard Tureck, and Luigi Mastroianni, Jr. 1985. "Psychological Evaluation and Support in a Program of In Vitro Fertilization and Embryo Transfer." *Fertility and Sterility* 43(1):48–53.

Friedler, Shevach, Linda C. Giudice, and Emmet J. Lamb. 1988. "Cryopreservation of Embryos and Ova." *Fertility and Sterility* 49 (5):743–761.

Friedman, J. M. 1974. "Legal Implications for Amniocentesis." *University of Pennsylvania Law Review* 123:149–195.

Fuchs, Victor R., and Leslie Perreault. 1986. "Expenditures for Reproduction-Related Health Care." *JAMA* 255:76.

Furrow, Barry R. 1984. "Surrogate Motherhood: A New Option for Parenting? *Law, Medicine and Health Care* (June), p. 106.

Genetic Technology News. 1986. "Market for DNA Probe Tests for Genetic Diseases." *Genetic Technology News* (November):6–7.

Glass, Bentley. 1975. "Ethical Problems Raised by Genetics." In Charles Birch and P. Albrecht, eds., *Genetics and the Quality of Life*. Australia: Pergamon Press.

Golbus, Michael S., et al. 1979. "Prenatal Genetic Diagnosis in 3000 Amniocenteses." *New England Journal of Medicine* 300:157–163.

Gold, Michael. 1985. "The Baby Makers." *Science* 85, April, pp. 26–38.

Golding, Martin P. 1968. "Ethical Issues in Biological Engineering." *UCLA Law Review* 15:443–479.

Goldsmith, Marsha F. 1988. "Trial Appears to Confirm Safety of Chorionic Villus Sampling Procedure." *JAMA* 259(24):3521–3522.

Gorovitz, Samuel 1978. "In Vitro Fertilization: Sense and Nonsense." Paper prepared for the Ethics Advisory Board. Appendix 3.

Gracia, Diego. 1988. "Spain: New Problems, New Books." *Hastings Center Report* 18(4):Supp. 28–29.

Green, Harold P. 1976. "Law and Genetic Control: Public Policy Questions." *Annals of the New York Academy of Sciences* 265(January):170–177.

Grobstein, Clifford. 1982. "The Moral Uses of 'Spare' Embryos." *Hastings Center Report* 12(3):5–6.

Grobstein, Clifford and Michael Flower. 1984. "Gene Therapy: Proceed With Caution." *Hastings Center Report* 14(2):13–17.

Grumbach, Melvin N. 1988. "Growth Hormone Therapy and the Short End of the Stick." *New England Journal of Medicine* 319(4):238–240.

Gustafson, James M. 1974. "Genetic Screening and Human Values." In Daniel Bergsma, ed., *Ethical, Social, and Legal Dimensions of Screening for Human Genetic Disease*. New York: Stratton.

Harris, L. E. 1981. "Artificial Insemination and Surrogate Motherhood—A Nursery Full of Unresolved Questions." *Willamette Law Review* 17:913–952.

Harsanyi, Zsolt, and Richard Hutton. 1981. *Genetic Prophecy: Beyond the Double Helix*. New York: Rawson, Wade Publishers, Inc.

Hartigan, Richard S. 1987. *The Future Remembered: An Essay in Biopolitics*. South Bend: University of Notre Dame Press.

Hartley, S. F., and L. M. Pietracyzk. 1979. "Preselecting the Sex of Offspring: Technologies, Attitudes and Implications." *Social Biology* 26(3):232–246.

Harvard Law Review. 1985. "Reproductive Technology and the Procreation Rights of the Unmarried." *Harvard Law Review* 98(3):669–685.

Henry, Alice et al. 1980. "Reversing Female Sterilization." *Population Reports* C-8: September.

Hewitt, Maria, and Neil A. Holtzman. 1988. "The Commercial Development of Tests for Human Genetic Disorders." Staff paper for Office of Technology Assessment.

Hippocrates. 1988. "Choices of the Heart." *Hippocrates* 2(3):40–41.

Hobbins, John C. 1988. "Selective Reduction—A Perinatal Necessity? *New England Journal of Medicine* 318(16):1062–1063.

Holden, Constance. 1982. "Looking at Genes in the Workplace." *Science* 217:336–337.

Holman, H. R., and D. B. Dutton. 1978. "A Case for Public Participation in Science Policy Formation and Practice." *Southern California Law Review* 51:1505, 1513–1514.

Howard, Ted, and Jeremy Rifkin. 1977. *Who Should Play God?* New York: Dell Publishing Company.

Hrdy, Sarah B. et al. 1988. "Daughters or Sons?" *Natural History* 97(April):63–82.

Hubbard, Ruth. 1980. "Test-Tube Babies: Solution or Problem?" *Technology Review* (March-April), pp. 10–12.

——1982. "Some Legal and Policy Implications of Recent Advances in Prenatal Diagnosis and Fetal Therapy." *Women's Rights Law Reporter* 7(3):201–218.

——1985. "Prenatal Diagnosis and Eugenic Ideology." *Women's Studies International Forum* 8(6):567–576.

Hubbard, Ruth, and Mary S. Henifin. 1985. "Genetic Screening of Prospective Parents and of Workers: Some Scientific and Social Issues." *International Journal of Health Services* 15(2):231–251.

Hughes, A. L. 1981. "Female Infanticide: Sex Ratio Manipulation in Humans." *Ethology and Sociobiology* 2:109–111.

Huxley, Aldous 1946. *Brave New World*. 2nd. ed. New York: Harper and Row.

Iizuka, R. et al. 1968. "The Physical and Mental Development of Children Born Following Artificial Insemination." *International Journal of Fertility* 13:24–32.

Isaacs, Stephen L., and Renee J. Holt. 1987. "Redefining Procreation: Facing the Issues." *Population Bulletin* 42(3):1–37.

Jonas, Hans. 1984. *The Imperative of Responsibility: In Search of an Ethics for the Technological Age*. Chicago: University of Chicago Press.

Jones, M. V. 1971. *A Technology Assessment Methodology. Vol. 1. Some Basic Propositions*. Washington, D.C.: MITRE Corporation.

Kass, Leon R. 1971. "The New Biology: What Price Relieving Man's Estate?" *Science* 174, November:779–788.

—— 1972. "Making Babies—the New Biology and the 'Old' Morality." *Public Interest* 26 (Winter):18–56.

—— 1976. "Implications of Prenatal Diagnosis for the Human Right to Life." In J.M. Humber and R.F. Almeder, eds., *Biomedical Ethics and the Law*. New York: Plenum Press.

—— 1981. " 'Making Babies' Revisited." In T.A. Shannon, ed., *Bioethics* 2nd ed. Ramsey, N.J.: Paulist Press.

Katz, B. F. 1978. "Legal Implications of In Vitro Fertilization and Its Regulation." Paper prepared for Ethics Advisory Board.

Keane, Noel P. 1980. "Legal Problems of Surrogate Motherhood." *Southern Illinois University Law Journal* 1980:147.

Keane, Noel P. and D. L. Breo. 1981. *The Surrogate Mother*. New York: Everest House.

Keeton, Kathy, and Yvonne Baskin. 1985. *Women of Tomorrow*. New York: St. Martin's Press.

Kern, Patricia A., and Kathleen M. Ridolfi. 1982. "The Fourteenth Amendment's Protection of a Woman's Right to Be a Single Parent through Artificial Insemination by Donor." *Women's Rights Law Reporter* 7(3):251–284.

Kevles, Daniel J. 1985. *In the Name of Eugenics: Genetics and the Use of Human Heredity*. Berkeley: University of California Press.

Kieffer, George H. 1975. *Ethical Issues in the Life Sciences*. New York: American Association for the Advancement of Science.

King, Patricia A. 1986. "Reproductive Technologies." *Biolaw*. Vol. 1. Frederick, Md.: University Publications of America.

Klass, Perri. 1989. "The Perfect Baby?" *The New York Times Magazine*, January 29, pp. 45–46.

Kolata, Gina. 1986a. "Manic-Depression: Is It Inherited?" *Science* 232(May 2):575–576.

—— 1986b. "Genetic Screening Raises Questions for Employers and Insurers." *Science* 232(April 18):317–319.

—— 1986c. "Researchers Hunt for Alzheimer's Disease Gene." *Science* 232(April 25):448–450.

—— 1986d. "Researchers Seek Melanoma Gene." *Science* 232(May 9):708–709.

Kotulak, Ronald. 1980. "Scientific Gains Being Used Against Women, Panel Says." *Chicago Tribune*, January 7, Sec. 1, p. 3.

Lancaster, Paul A. L. 1985. "Obstetric Outcome." In C. Wood and A. Trounson, eds., *Clinics in Obstetrics and Gynaecology: New Clinical Issues in In Vitro Fertilization*. London: W. B. Saunders.

Lantos, John, Mark Siegler, and Leona Cuttler. 1989. "Ethical Issues in Growth Hormone Therapy." *JAMA* 261 (7):1020–1024.

Lappé, Marc. 1972. "Moral Obligations and the Fallacies of 'Genetic Control.'" *Theological Studies* 33 (September):411–427.

Lappé, Marc, and P. A. Martin. 1978. "The Place of the Public in the Conduct of Science." *Southern California Law Review* 52:1535–1539.

Lewin, Roger. 1987. "National Academy Looks at Human Genome Project, Sees Progress," *Science* 235:747–748.

Lewis, Ricki. 1987. "Genetic-Marker Testing: Are We Ready for It?" *Issues in Science and Technology* 4(1):76–82.

Lieber, James. 1989. "A Piece of Yourself in the World." *The Atlantic Monthly* (June), pp. 76–80.

Lieberman, E. J. 1968. "A Doctor Forecasts Determining of Sex of Child in Advance." *New York Times* (November 27):27.

Lippmann, Walter. 1945. *The Public Philosophy*. Boston: Little, Brown.

Lorber, John. 1987. "Gender Politics and In Vitro Fertilization Use." *Women and Health*.

Lowi, Ted J. 1969. *The End of Liberalism*. New York: W. W. Norton.

Lowrance, William W. 1982. "Choosing Our Pleasures and Our Poisons: Risk Assessment for the 1980s." In A.H. Teich and R. Thornton, eds., *Science, Technology, and the Issues of the Eighties: Policy Outlook*. Boulder: Westview Press.

Macri, James N., and Robert R. Weiss. 1982. "Prenatal Serum Alpha-Fetoprotein Screening for Neural Tube Defects." *Obstetrics and Gynecology* 59(5):633.

Mady, T. M. 1981. "Surrogate Mothers: The Legal Issues." *American Journal of Law and Medicine* 7(3):323–352.

Main, Denise M., and Michael T. Mennuti. 1986. "Neural Tube Defects: Issues in Prenatal Diagnosis and Counselling." *Obstetrics and Gynecology* 67(1):1–16.

Marx, Jean L. 1986. "Gene Therapy—So Near Yet So Far Away." *Science* 232(May 16):824–825.

——1988. "Eye Cancer Gene Linked to New Malignancies." *Science* 241(July 1):293–294.

Matthewman, William D. 1984. "Title VII and Genetic Testing: Can Your Genes Screen You Out of a Job?" *Howard Law Journal* 27(Fall):1185–1224.

Mathieu, Deborah. 1984. "The Baby Doe Controversy." *Arizona State Law Journal* 1984(4):602–626.

Medawar, Peter B. 1969. "The Genetic Improvement of Man." *Australian Annals of Medicine* 4:317–320.

Medical Research International. 1988. "In Vitro Fertilization/Embryo Transfer in the United States: 1985 and 1986 Results from the National IVF/ET Registry." *Fertility and Sterility* 49(2):212–215.

Mies, Maria. 1987. "Sexist and Racist Implications of New Reproductive Technologies." *Alternatives* 12:323–342.

Milbrath, Lester W. 1986. "A Governance Structure Designed to Help a Society Learn How to Become Sustainable." Paper presented to the annual meeting of the American Political Science Association, August 30, Washington, D.C.

Miller, Jon D. 1989. Personal communication on status of national scientific literacy study.

Miller, Jon D. et al. 1980. *Citizenship in an Age of Science: Changing Attitudes Among Young Adults*. New York: Pergamon Press.

Miller, R. 1983. "Surrogate Parenting: An Infant Industry Presents Society With Legal, Ethical Questions." *Obstetrics and Gynecological News* 3:15–19.

Milunsky, Aubrey. 1977. *Know Your Genes*. Boston: Houghten-Mifflin.

Monroe, Alan D. 1975. *Public Opinion in America*. New York: Dodd, Mead

Motulsky, Arno G., and Jeffrey Murray. 1983. "Will Prenatal Diagnosis with Selective Abortion Affect Society's Attitude Toward the Handicapped?" In Kare Berg and Knut E. Tranoy, eds., *Research Ethics*, pp. 227–291. New York: Alan R. Liss.

Muller, Hermann J. 1961. "Human Evolution by Voluntary Choice of Germ Plasm." *Science* 134:643–649.

Murphy, E. A., G. Chase, and A. Rodriguez. 1978. "Genetic Intervention: Some Social, Psychological, and Philosophical Aspects." In B. H. Cohen et al., eds., *Genetic Issues in Public Health and Medicine*. Springfield, Ill.: Charles C. Thomas.

Nakamura, Robert T., and Frank Smallwood. 1980. *The Politics of Policy Implementation*. New York: St. Martin's Press.

National Academy of Sciences. 1975. Genetic Screening: Programs, Principles, and Research. Washington, D.C.: National Academy Press.

National University Hospital. 1989. "World's First." *Lifeline* 3(July):1.

Nelkin, D. 1980. "Science and Technology Policy and the Democratic Process." In *Five Year Outlook*. Vol. 12. Washington, D.C.: National Science Foundation.

Nelson, Lawrence J., and Nancy Millikin. 1988. "Compelled Medical Treatment of Pregnant Women: Life, Liberty, and Law in Conflict." *JAMA* 259(7)1060–1066.

New York State Task Force on Life and the Law. 1988. *Surrogate Parenting: Analysis and Recommendations for Public Policy*.

New Zealand, Law Reform Division. 1986. *New Birth Technologies: A Summary of Submissions Received on the Issues Paper*. Wellington, N.Z.: Department of Justice.

Nolan, Kathleen, and Sara Swenson. 1988. "New Tools, New Dilemmas: Genetic Frontiers." *Hastings Center Report* 18(5):40–46.

Oakley, Ann. 1984. *The Captured Womb: A History of the Medical Care of Pregnant Women*. Oxford: Oxford Press.

Office of Medical Applications of Research, National Institutes of Health. 1984. "The Use of Diagnostic Ultrasound Imaging During Pregnancy." *JAMA* 252(5):669–672.

Office of Technology Assessment. 1981. *Impacts of Applied Genetics: Micro-*

Organisms, Plants, and Animals. Washington, D.C.: U.S. Government Printing Office.

——1987. *OTA Proposal: Infertility Prevention and Treatment.* Washington, D.C.: OTA.

——1988. *Infertility: Medical and Social Choices.* Washington, D.C.: U.S. Government Printing Office.

——1988a. *Mapping Our Genes: Genome Projects: How Big, How Fast?* Washington, D.C.: U.S. Government Printing Office.

——1988b. *Artificial Insemination: Practice in the United States.* Washington, D.C.: U.S. Government Printing Office.

Olson, Steve. 1986. *Biotechnology: An Industry Comes of Age.* Washington, D.C.: National Academy Press.

Organization for Economic Cooperation and Development. 1981. *Science and Technology Policy for the 1980s.* Paris: OECD.

Overall, Christine. 1987. *Ethics and Human Reproduction: A Feminist Analysis.* Boston: Allen and Unwin.

Pareto, V. 1935. *The Mind and Society.* New York: Harcourt, Brace and Company.

Parker, Philip. 1983. "Motivation of Surrogate Mothers: Initial Findings." *American Journal of Psychiatry* 140(1):115–118.

Partington, M. W. 1986. "X-Linked Mental Retardation: Caveats in Genetic Counseling." *American Journal of Medical Genetics* 23(1–2):101–109.

Perry, Tracy B. 1985. "Fetoscopy." *Progress in Clinical and Biological Research* 163B:207–212.

Petchesky, Rosalind P. 1980. "Reproductive Freedom: Beyond a Woman's Right to Choose." *Signs: Journal of Women in Culture and Society* 5:661–685.

Philip, J., and J. Bang. 1985. "Prenatal Diagnosis in Multiple Gestations." In Karen Filkins and Joseph F. Russo, eds., *Human Prenatal Diagnosis.* New York: Marcel Dekker.

President's Commission for the Study of Ethical Problems in Medicine and Biomedical and Behavioral Research. 1982. *Splicing Life: the Social and Ethical Issues of Genetic Engineering with Human Beings.* Washington, D.C.: U.S. Government Printing Office.

——1983. *Screening and Counseling for Genetic Conditions.* Washington, D.C.: U.S. Government Printing Office.

Price, David K. 1978. "Endless Frontier or Bureaucratic Morass?" *Daedalus* 107(2):75–92.

Purdy, L. M. 1978. "Genetic Diseases: Can Having Children Be Immoral." In J. J. Buckley, ed., *Genetics Now: Ethical Issues in Genetic Research.* Washington: University Press of America.

Quinlan, R. William, Amelia C. Cruz, and John F. Huddleston. 1986. "Sonographic Detection of Urinary-Tract Anomalies." *Obstetrics and Gynecology* 67(2):558–570.

Ramsey, Paul. 1975. *The Ethics of Fetal Research*. New Haven: Yale University Press.

Rawlins, R. G., Z. Binor, E. Radwanska, and W. P. Dmowski. 1988. "Microsurgical Enucleation of Tripronuclear Human Zygotes." *Fertility and Sterility* 50(2):266–271.

Raymond, Chris Anne. 1988. "In Vitro Fertilization Enters Stormy Adolescence as Experts Debate the Odds." *JAMA* 259(4):464–466.

Reilly, Philip. 1977. *Genetics, Law and Social Policy*. Cambridge: Harvard University Press.

Rettig, F. A. 1982. "Applying Science and Technology to Public Purposes: A Synthesis." In A.H. Teich and R. Thornton, eds., *Science, Technology, and the Issues of the Eighties; Policy Outlook*. Boulder: Westview Press.

Rhoden, Nancy K. and John D. Arras. 1985. "Withholding Treatment from Baby Doe: From Discrimination to Child Abuse." *Milbank Memorial Fund Quarterly* 63(1):18–51.

Ribes, B. 1978. *Biology and Ethics*. New York: UNESCO.

Roberts, Leslie. 1988. "Race for Cystic Fibrosis Gene Nears End." *Science* 240(April 15):282–284.

Robertson, John A. 1983. "Procreative Liberty and the Control of Conception, Pregnancy, and Childbirth." *Virginia Law Review* 69 (3):405–464.

Rodriguez, Helen. 1980. "Concluding Remarks: Depo-Provera and Sterilization Abuse." In Helen B. Holmes et al., eds., *Birth Control and Controlling Birth: Women-Centered Perspectives*. Clifton, N.J.: Humana Press.

Rosettenstein, D. S. 1981. "Defining a Parent: The New Biology and the Rebirth of Filius Nullius." *New Law Journal* 131:1095–1096.

Rothman, Barbara Katz. 1986. *The Tentative Pregnancy: Prenatal Diagnosis and the Future of Motherhood*. New York: Viking.

——1987. "Surrogacy: A Question of Values." *Conscience* 8(3):1–15.

Rothschild, Joan, ed. 1983. *Machina ex Dea: Feminist Perspectives in Technology*. New York: Pergamon Press.

Rowland, Robyn. 1985. "The Social and Psychological Consequences of Secrecy in Artificial Insemination by Donor (AID) Programmes." *Social Sciences and Medicine* 21(4):391–396.

——1985a. "A Child at Any Price?" *Women's Studies International Forum* 8(6):539–546.

Schacter, Julius, and Mary-Ann Shafer. 1985. "Female Adolescents with Chlamydia: Tomorrow's Candidates for In Vitro Fertilization?" *Western Journal of Medicine* 143(1):100.

Schoenberg, B. 1979. "Science and Anti-Science in Confrontation." *Man and Medicine* 4(2):79–102.

Schwartz, D., and M. J. Mayaux. 1982. "Female Fecundity as a Function of Age." *New England Journal of Medicine* 306:404–406.

Scott, David C. 1989. "Curb on Test-Tube Baby Research Roils Assuie Scientisits." *The Christian Science Monitor* (April 17), p. 4.

Scriver, Charles R. et al. 1985. "Population Screening: Report of a Workshop." *Progress in Clinical and Biological Research* 163B:89–152.

Seibel, Machelle M. 1988. "A New Era in Reproductive Technology." *New England Journal of Medicine* 318(13)828–834.

Selden, Richard F., Marek J. Skoskiewicz, Paul S. Russell, and Howard M. Goodman. 1987. "Regulation of Insulin-Gene Expression: Implications for Gene Therapy." *New England Journal of Medicine* 317(17):1067–1075.

Sellors, John W., James B. Mahony, Max A. Chernesky, and Darlyne J. Rath. 1988. "Tubal Factor Infertility: An Association with Prior Chlamydial Infection and Asymptomatic Salpingitis." *Fertility and Sterility* 49(3):451–456.

Sewell, Sandra S. 1980. "Sterilization Abuse and Hispanic Women." In Helen B. Holmes et al., eds., *Birth Control and Controlling Birth: Women-Centered Perspectives.* Clifton, N.J.: Humana Press.

Shaman, J. M. 1980. "Legal Aspects of Artificial Insemination." *Journal of Family Law* 18:330–346.

Shaw, Margery W. 1978. "Genetically Defective Children: Emerging Legal Considerations." *American Journal of Law and Medicine* 3:336–349.

Sherman, J. K. 1980. "Historical Synopsis of Human Semen Cryobanking." In G. David and W. S. Price, eds., *Human Artificial Insemination and Semen Preservation.* New York: Plenum Press.

Shick, Alan. 1977. "Complex Policy Making in the United States Senate." In *Policy Analyses on Major Issues prepared for the Commission on the Operation of the Senate.* Washington, D.C.: U.S. Government Printing Office.

Short, Robert V. 1978. "Human In Vitro Fertilization and Embryo Transfer." Paper prepared for Ethics Advisory Board.

Simpson, Joe Leigh. 1986. "Methods for Detecting Neural Tube Defects." *Contemporary OB/GYN* 1986:202–222.

Sivin, I. 1982. "The NORPLANT Contraceptive Method: A Report on Three Years of Use." *Studies in Family Planning* 13:258–262.

Skolnikoff, Eugene B. 1982. "Science, Technology and International Security: A Synthesis." In A.H. Teich and R. Thornton, eds., *Science, Technology, and the Issues of the Eighties: Policy Outlook.* Boulder: Westview Press.

Snowden, Robert, G. D. Mitchell, and E. M. Snowden. 1983. *Artificial Reproduction.* London: George Allen and Unwin, Ltd.

Sorenson, J. R. 1974. "Some Social and Psychologic Issues in Genetic Screening." In D. Bergsma, ed., *Ethical, Social and Legal Dimensions of Screening for Human Genetic Disease.* New York: Stratton.

Steinbrook, Robert. 1986. "In California, Voluntary Mass Prenatal Screening." *Hastings Center Report* 16(5):5–7.

Stich, Stephen P. 1983. "The Genetic Adventure." *Report from the Center for Philosophy and Public Policy* 3(2):9–12.

Toth, C., D. Washington, and O. Davies. 1987. "Reimbursement for In Vitro Fertilization: A Survey of HIAA Companies." *Research and Statistical Bulletin.* Washington, D.C.: Health Insurance Association of America.

Tranoy, Knut Erik. 1988. "Biomedical Value Conflict." *Hastings Center Report* 18(4): Supp. 8–10.

Tribe, Lawrence H. 1973. "Technology Assessment and the Fourth Discontinuity: The Limits of Instrumental Rationality." *Southern California Law Review* 46 (June):617–660.

Trotzig, M. A. 1980. "The Defective Child and the Actions for Wrongful Life and Wrongful Birth." *Family Law Quarterly* 14:16–18.

Twiss, Summer B. 1974. "Ethical Issues in Genetic Screening: Models of Genetic Responsibility." In D. Bergsma, ed., *Ethical, Social and Legal Dimensions of Screening for Human Genetic Disease*. New York: Stratton.

U.S. Congress, House of Representatives. 1987a. Select Committee on Children, Youth, and Families, Hearing on "Alternative Reproductive Technologies: Implications for Children and Families." Washington, D.C.: U.S. Government Printing Office.

——1987b. Subcommittee on Civil Service, Committee on Post Office and Civil Service, Hearing on "Federal Employee Family-Building Act of 1987." Washington, D.C.: U.S. Government Printing Office.

——1988. Subcommittee on Regulation and Business Opportunities, Committee on Small Business, Hearing on "Consumer Protection Issues Involving In Vitro Fertilization Centers." Washington, D.C.: U.S. Government Printing Office.

van Regenmorter, J., S. van Regenmorter, and J. S. McIlhaney, Jr. 1986. *Dear God, Why Can't We Have a Baby?* Grand Rapids: Baker Book House.

Veit, Christina R., and Raphael Jewelawicz. 1988. "Gender Preselection: Facts and Myths." *Fertility and Sterility* 49(6):937–940.

Verp, Marion S., and Joe Leigh Simpson. 1985. "Amniocentesis for Cytogenetic Studies." In Karen Filkins and Joseph F. Russo, eds., *Human Prenatal Diagnosis*, pp. 13–41. New York: Marcel Dekker.

Wald, P. M. 1975. "Basic Personal and Civil Rights: Principal Paper." In President's Committee on Mental Retardation, *The Mentally Retarded Citizen and the Law*. New York: The Free Press.

Walters, William A. W., and Peter Singer. 1982. *Test-Tube Babies*. Melbourne: Oxford University Press.

Warsof, Steven L. et al. 1986. "Routine Ultrasound Screening for Antenatal Detection of Intrauterine Growth Retardation." *Obstetrics and Gynecology* 67(1):33–38.

Webber, David J. 1986. "Analyzing Political Feasibility: Political Scientists' Unique Contribution to Policy Analysis." *Policy Studies Journal* 14(4):545–549.

Weiner, Charles. 1982. "Relations of Science, Government and Industry: The Case of Recombinant DNA." In A.H. Teich and R. Thornton, eds., *Science, Technology, and the Issues of the Eighties: Policy Outlook*. Boulder: Westview Press.

Wenk, Edward. 1981. "Political Limits in Steering Technology." In A. H. Teich, ed. *Technology and Man's Future*. New York: St. Martin's Press.

Wertz, Dorothy C., and John C. Fletcher. 1989. "Fatal Knowledge? Prenatal Diagnosis and Sex Selection." *Hastings Center Report* 19(3)21–27.

Williams, P., and G. Stevens. 1982. "What Now for Test Tube Babies?" *New Scientist* 93(129):312–317.

Wimberley, Edward T. 1982. "The RSP Method of Tubal Occlusion: A Review and Update." *Biomedical Bulletin* 3(1):1–6.

Winslade, William J. 1981. "Surrogate Mothers: Private Right or Public Wrong?" *Journal of Medical Ethics* 7:153–154.

Woliver, Laura R. 1989. "New Reproductive Technologies: Challenges to Women's Control of Gestation and Birth." In Robert H. Blank and Miriam K. Mills, eds., *Biomedical Technology and Public Policy*. New York: Greenwood Press.

Zaneveld, Lourens J. D., James W. Burns, Stan Beyler, William Depel, and Seymour Shapiro. 1988. "Development of a Potentially Reversible Vas Deferens Occlusion Device and Evaluation in Primates." *Fertility and Sterility* 49(3):527–533.

INDEX

CASES INDEX

271